Learning to Diagnose with Simulations

Frank Fischer • Ansgar Opitz
Editors

Learning to Diagnose with Simulations

Examples from Teacher Education and Medical Education

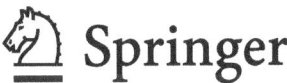

Editors
Frank Fischer
Chair of Education and Educational
Psychology
Department of Psychology, LMU Munich
Munich, Germany

Ansgar Opitz
Chair of Education and Educational
Psychology
Department of Psychology, LMU Munich
Munich, Germany

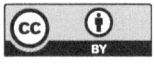

ISBN 978-3-030-89146-6   ISBN 978-3-030-89147-3 (eBook)
https://doi.org/10.1007/978-3-030-89147-3

© The Editor(s) (if applicable) and The Author(s) 2022. This book is an open access publication.
Open Access This book is licensed under the terms of the Creative Commons Attribution 4.0 International License (http://creativecommons.org/licenses/by/4.0/), which permits use, sharing, adaptation, distribution and reproduction in any medium or format, as long as you give appropriate credit to the original author(s) and the source, provide a link to the Creative Commons license and indicate if changes were made.
The images or other third party material in this book are included in the book's Creative Commons license, unless indicated otherwise in a credit line to the material. If material is not included in the book's Creative Commons license and your intended use is not permitted by statutory regulation or exceeds the permitted use, you will need to obtain permission directly from the copyright holder.
The use of general descriptive names, registered names, trademarks, service marks, etc. in this publication does not imply, even in the absence of a specific statement, that such names are exempt from the relevant protective laws and regulations and therefore free for general use.
The publisher, the authors and the editors are safe to assume that the advice and information in this book are believed to be true and accurate at the date of publication. Neither the publisher nor the authors or the editors give a warranty, expressed or implied, with respect to the material contained herein or for any errors or omissions that may have been made. The publisher remains neutral with regard to jurisdictional claims in published maps and institutional affiliations.

This Springer imprint is published by the registered company Springer Nature Switzerland AG
The registered company address is: Gewerbestrasse 11, 6330 Cham, Switzerland

Contents

1 **Learning to Diagnose with Simulations: Introduction** 1
Frank Fischer, Olga Chernikova, and Ansgar Opitz

2 **A Theoretical Framework for Fostering Diagnostic Competences with Simulations in Higher Education** 5
Olga Chernikova, Nicole Heitzmann, Ansgar Opitz, Tina Seidel, and Frank Fischer

3 **Learning to Diagnose Primary Students' Mathematical Competence Levels and Misconceptions in Document-Based Simulations** 17
Angelika Wildgans-Lang, Sarah Scheuerer, Andreas Obersteiner, Frank Fischer, and Kristina Reiss

4 **Diagnosing Mathematical Argumentation Skills: A Video-Based Simulation for Pre-Service Teachers** 33
Elias Codreanu, Sina Huber, Sarah Reinhold, Daniel Sommerhoff, Birgit J. Neuhaus, Ralf Schmidmaier, Stefan Ufer, and Tina Seidel

5 **Diagnosing 6th Graders' Understanding of Decimal Fractions: Fostering Mathematics Pre-Service Teachers' Diagnostic Competences with Simulated One-on-One Interviews** 49
Bernhard Marczynski, Larissa J. Kaltefleiter, Matthias Siebeck, Christof Wecker, Kathleen Stürmer, and Stefan Ufer

6 **Diagnosing the Instructional Quality of Biology Lessons Based on Staged Videos: Developing DiKoBi, A Video-Based Simulation** 63
Maria Kramer, Julia Stürmer, Christian Förtsch, Tina Seidel, Stefan Ufer, Martin R. Fischer, and Birgit J. Neuhaus

7	Learning to Diagnose Secondary School Students' Scientific Reasoning Skills in Physics and Biology: Video-Based Simulations for Pre-Service Teachers	83
	Amadeus J. Pickal, Christof Wecker, Birgit J. Neuhaus, and Raimund Girwidz	
8	Learning to Diagnose Students' Behavioral, Developmental, and Learning Disorders in a Simulation-Based Learning Environment for Pre-Service Teachers	97
	Elisabeth Bauer, Michael Sailer, Jan Kiesewetter, Claudia Schulz, Iryna Gurevych, Martin R. Fischer, and Frank Fischer	
9	Live and Video Simulations of Medical History-Taking: Theoretical Background, Design, Development, and Validation of a Learning Environment	109
	Maximilian C. Fink, Victoria Reitmeier, Matthias Siebeck, Frank Fischer, and Martin R. Fischer	
10	Diagnosing Collaboratively: A Theoretical Model and a Simulation-Based Learning Environment	123
	Anika Radkowitsch, Michael Sailer, Martin R. Fischer, Ralf Schmidmaier, and Frank Fischer	
11	Conclusions and Outlook: Toward more Systematic Research on the Use of Simulations in Higher Education	143
	Ansgar Opitz, Martin R. Fischer, Tina Seidel, and Frank Fischer	

Index 151

Chapter 1
Learning to Diagnose with Simulations: Introduction

Frank Fischer, Olga Chernikova, and Ansgar Opitz

Making decisions require professionals in different fields to be able to identify, understand, and even predict situations and events relevant to their professions. This makes diagnosis an essential part of professional competences across domains. Diagnosis involves identifying the problem, analyzing the context, and application of obtained knowledge and experience to make practical decisions.

Scientific understanding of diagnostic competences improved significantly in the past years, and a range of measurement tools emerged (Herppich et al., 2018; Loibl et al., 2020). The existing empirical evidence supports the claim that problem-solving facilitates complex skills in different domains (Belland et al., 2017; Dochy et al., 2003). Problem-solving and reasoning in many domains rely on epistemic activities, for example, problem identification or collecting evidence (Fischer et al., 2014), which are also relevant for diagnosing. Simulation-based learning in turn, enables approximation of practice (Grossman et al., 2009) but also provides learning opportunities which are not present in real world situations (e.g., repeating a task over and over again to practice). Effectiveness of simulation-based learning also received empirical support with moderate to high effects on learning outcomes (e.g., in medical education, see Cook, 2014), however the question of how simulations can be designed to be most beneficial for students with different learning prerequisites has been addressed to a lesser extent (but see Chernikova et al., 2020) and remains largely open.

Two strands of research on diagnostic competences are particularly dynamic and promising, namely those in medical and teacher education. Although simulations are used in different areas of professional education, little research focuses on finding

F. Fischer (✉) · O. Chernikova · A. Opitz
Chair of Education and Educational Psychology, Department of Psychology, LMU Munich, Munich, Germany
e-mail: frank.fischer@psy.lmu.de

© The Author(s) 2022
F. Fischer, A. Opitz (eds.), *Learning to Diagnose with Simulations*,
https://doi.org/10.1007/978-3-030-89147-3_1

interdisciplinary commonalities and effective design features that can be transferred from one domain to another. We assume that medical and teacher education domains can learn a lot from each other with regard to the design of learning environments to foster the development of professional competencies (Heitzmann et al., 2019).

In this book, we present a coherent set of approaches to simulation-based learning of diagnostic competences across the domains of medical and teacher education. The coherency is achieved by measures on three levels.

First, the collection builds on a joint conceptual framework specifying learning prerequisites, learning process, instructional support, diagnostic context and diagnostic competences as the outcome, which will be introduced in Chap. 2. To elaborate on one exemplary of the framework's concepts, the simulations described in the chapters vary with respect to three main *contextual dimensions*. (1) They vary with respect to the domain and topics within the domains, e.g., fever of unknown origin in medicine or text comprehension problems in primary school in teacher education. (2) The diagnostic mode, that is whether the diagnostic processes is performed alone or together with one or more additional diagnosticians (e.g., an internist and a radiologist diagnosing the causes of a patient's fiver or a biology teacher and a physics teacher determining a secondary school student's scientific argumentation skill). The third dimension (3) refers to whether documents are the main information sources (e.g., X-ray pictures; student solutions of mathematical tasks) or whether the diagnostician need to dynamically interact with persons, e.g., a patient or a student. These variations within the common framework are necessary to address the heterogeneity of situations diagnosing practitioners will face.

Second, all of the chapters refer to the same basic definitions of diagnosing and diagnostic competences. Throughout this book, diagnosing is broadly defined "as the goal-oriented collection and interpretation of case-specific or problem-specific information to reduce uncertainty in order to make medical or educational decisions (Heitzmann et al., 2019, p. 4). Diagnostic competences are "individual dispositions enabling people to apply their knowledge in diagnostic activities according to professional standards to collect and interpret data in order to make high-quality decisions" (Heitzmann et al., 2019, p. 5).

Third, the individual Chaps. 3, 4, 5, 6, 7, 8, 9, and 10 in the collection position the reported work with respect to four overarching research questions. These are (1) What processes are central to generate desired learning outcomes in simulations aimed at diagnostic competences? (2) How can learners in simulations be supported to optimize learning outcomes? (3) Which variables mediate or moderate the effects of instructional support? (4) How can the simulations be adapted to fit the individual learners?

The order of the chapters is based on the different domains included. Chaps. 3, 4, and 5 report on simulations from mathematics education. Chaps. 6 and 7 present simulations in the context of science education. Chap. 8 describes a simulation in the psychology of teacher education in which future teachers learn to identify indicators of learning disorders in school students. Chaps. 9 and 10 are situated in medical education. Chap. 11 then offers a conclusion and an outlook which is focused on the four overarching research questions mentioned above.

The simulation-based learning environments presented in this book have been developed to enable learners to actively engage in diagnostic activities in different domains. They were validated, for example, by asking experts how authentic they consider the simulations to be in relation to real world environments, or by comparing the diagnostic activities and accuracies of novices and more knowledgeable learners, including experts. The simulations allow for investigating how students proceed in applying their different knowledge bases to diagnostic problems—and how their strategies differ from those of experts. In the future, they will enable research on the effects of instructional support in simulations. When different domains are included, the scientific knowledge on the instructional design of simulations for learning to diagnose could even be tested for generalizability across domains.

Acknowledgments The editors are thankful to Melissa James, Shabib Shaikh, and Helen van der Strelt at Springer Nature, and Alexa Krickel at LMU for their important contributions to coordinating the preparation and the publication of the book. The research presented in this chapter was funded by a grant from the Deutsche Forschungsgemeinschaft (DFG-FOR 2385).

References

Belland, B. R., Walker, A. E., Kim, N. J., & Lefler, M. (2017). Synthesizing results from empirical research on computer-based scaffolding in STEM education: A meta-analysis. *Review of Educational Research, 87*(2), 309–344. https://doi.org/10.3102/0034654316670999

Chernikova, O., Heitzmann, N., Stadler, M., Holzberger, D., Seidel, T., & Fischer, F. (2020). Simulation-based learning in higher education: A meta-analysis. *Review of Educational Research, 90*(4), 499–541.

Cook, D. A. (2014). How much evidence does it take? A cumulative meta-analysis of outcomes of simulation-based education. *Medical Education, 48*(8), 750–760. https://doi.org/10.1111/medu.12473

Dochy, F., Segers, M., Van den Bossche, P., & Gijbels, D. (2003). Effects of problem-based learning: A meta-analysis. *Learning and Instruction, 13*(5), 533–568.

Fischer, F., Kollar, I., Ufer, S., Sodian, B., Hussmann, H., Pekrun, R., et al. (2014). Scientific reasoning and argumentation: Advancing an interdisciplinary research agenda in education. *Frontline Learning Research, 2*(2), 28–45. https://doi.org/10.14786/flr.v2i2.96

Grossman, P., Hammerness, K., & McDonald, M. (2009). Redefining teaching, re-imagining teacher education. *Teachers and Teaching: Theory and Practice, 15*(2), 273–289.

Heitzmann, N., Seidel, T., Opitz, A., Hetmanek, A., Wecker, C., Fischer, M., Ufer, S., Schmidmaier, R., Neuhaus, B., Siebeck, M., Stürmer, K., Obersteiner, A., Reiss, K., Girwidz, R., & Fischer, F. (2019). Facilitating diagnostic competences in simulations: A conceptual framework and a research agenda for medical and teacher education. *Frontline Learning Research, 7*(4), 1–24. https://doi.org/10.14786/flr.v7i4.384

Herppich, S., Praetorius, A. K., Förster, N., Glogger-Frey, I., Karst, K., Leutner, D., ... Hetmanek, A. (2018). Teachers' assessment competence: Integrating knowledge-, process-, and product-oriented approaches into a competence-oriented conceptual model. *Teaching and Teacher Education, 76*, 181–193.

Loibl, K., Leuders, T., & Dörfler, T. (2020). A framework for explaining teachers' diagnostic judgements by cognitive modeling (DiacoM). *Teaching and Teacher Education, 91*, 103059.

Open Access This chapter is licensed under the terms of the Creative Commons Attribution 4.0 International License (http://creativecommons.org/licenses/by/4.0/), which permits use, sharing, adaptation, distribution and reproduction in any medium or format, as long as you give appropriate credit to the original author(s) and the source, provide a link to the Creative Commons license and indicate if changes were made.

The images or other third party material in this chapter are included in the chapter's Creative Commons license, unless indicated otherwise in a credit line to the material. If material is not included in the chapter's Creative Commons license and your intended use is not permitted by statutory regulation or exceeds the permitted use, you will need to obtain permission directly from the copyright holder.

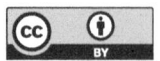

Chapter 2
A Theoretical Framework for Fostering Diagnostic Competences with Simulations in Higher Education

Olga Chernikova, Nicole Heitzmann, Ansgar Opitz, Tina Seidel, and Frank Fischer

2.1 Theoretical Overview

2.1.1 Instructional Support in Facilitating Competences

The conceptual framework used in this book is based on theoretical and empirical findings on skill development and theories of expertise development (Anderson, 1983; Jonassen, 1997; Renkl & Atkinson, 2003; Van Lehn, 1996), which suggests that learners need sufficient prior knowledge and to engage in complex practice opportunities to improve their professional competencies. Existing research on complex learning environments supports the claim that learning is more effective when instructional support is included (Lazonder & Harmsten, 2016). One possibility to avoid ineffective learning related to exposure to complex and ill-structured problems, particularly at early stages of expertise development, is to accompany the challenging tasks with scaffolding procedures, particularly those emphasizing metacognition and reflection as the main mechanisms of learning through experience. Therefore, we also include an overview of scaffolding types and measures as part of our theoretical framework.

O. Chernikova (✉) · N. Heitzmann · A. Opitz · F. Fischer
Chair of Education and Educational Psychology, Department of Psychology, LMU Munich, Munich, Germany
e-mail: o.chernikova@psy.lmu.de

T. Seidel
Friedl Schöller Endowed Chair for Educational Psychology, School of Education, Technical University of Munich (TUM), Munich, Germany

2.1.2 Simulations in Medical and Teacher Education

A simulation is a model or representation of reality (object, system, or situation) with certain parameters that can be controlled or manipulated. The aim of a simulation is to arrive at a better understanding of the interconnections between the variables in the system or to put different strategies to test (Frasson & Blanchard, 2012; Shannon, 1975; Wissenschaftsrat., 2014). Thus, a central goal of simulations teaching diagnostic competences is to provide training opportunities in which learners can take diagnostic actions on cases with a certain similarity to professional practice (Seidel et al., 2015; Shavelson, 2013). Both digital simulations and face-to-face role-plays have been used as simulation-based learning environments. Numerous primary research on the effectiveness of simulations in medical and teacher education supports their effectiveness (e.g., Koparan & Yılmaz, 2015; Liaw et al., 2010; Matsuda et al., 2013). Meta-analytic studies in medical education (e.g., Cook et al., 2012, 2013) provide evidence supporting the generalizability of the high effects of simulations. However, the open question is what features and parameters make simulations most effective in different contexts for learners with certain personal characteristics, such as learning prerequisites, different levels of prior professional knowledge, and levels of expertise.

2.2 Model Description

The conceptual model (Fig. 2.1) consists of five essential blocks of elements:

"Test performance" block: diagnostic competences are considered to be the target learning outcome and can be measured by assessing the efficiency and the accuracy of the diagnosis, applying professional knowledge, and performing appropriate diagnostic activities.

"Processes in simulation-based learning environments" block: activities in simulation-based learning environments are hypothesized to directly affect the learning outcomes. This block also includes diagnostic activities performed to acquire the target knowledge and competences and an intermediate assessment of the diagnostic accuracy and efficiency during the learning phase.

"Individual learning prerequisites" block: the following factors are hypothesized to have (1) a direct effect on the development of diagnostic competences as learning outcomes and (2) an indirect effect via Block II by specifying the way learning strategies and instructional support are utilized. This block includes the existing professional knowledge base: learners' conceptual and strategic knowledge, executive functions/working memory capacity, motivational variables, and interest.

"Instructional support" block: instructions include different types of scaffolding and ways to present information to the learners. They are hypothesized to influence the improvement of diagnostic competences by supporting learning processes and activities. The availability of appropriate instructional support that matches the

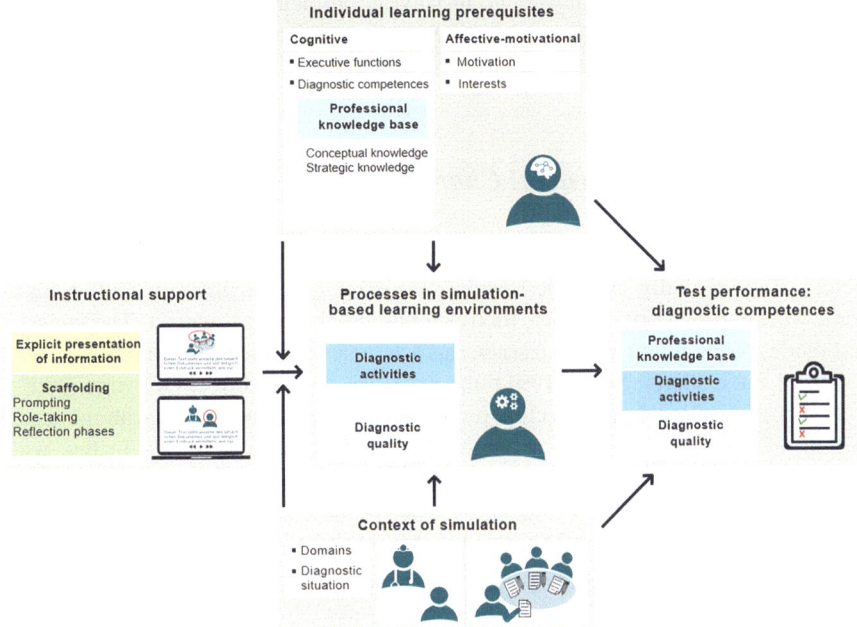

Fig. 2.1 Fostering diagnostic competences with simulation-based learning: adapted from conceptual framework by the COSIMA research unit (Heitzmann et al., 2019)

learning goals and learners' individual prerequisites determines the effectiveness of simulation-based learning environments.

The "Context of simulation" block encompasses the construction of learning environments and competence assessments and is hypothesized to have an effect on learning processes, the types of instructional support that can be utilized, and outcomes. This block includes the domain and the nature of the diagnostic situation (the information base and the need to collaborate during the diagnosis).

In the following paragraphs, we will describe the specific variables included in the five blocks of the conceptual model in more detail.

2.2.1 Professional Knowledge Base

The definition and differentiation of knowledge types constituting the professional knowledge base in the model are adopted from previous research in teacher and medical education (Förtsch et al., 2018). Professional knowledge consists of content and strategic knowledge. Content knowledge as defined by Shulman (1987) or conceptual knowledge (Stark et al., 2011) refers to the knowledge of subject matter, key terms, and their interrelations. Strategic knowledge, in turn, relates to the application of conceptual knowledge to solve a problem. The distinction between strategical and conceptual knowledge has been validated in empirical studies in medical education and beyond (e.g., Förtsch et al., 2018).

2.2.2 Individual Learners' Characteristics

Apart from the prior professional knowledge base, a range of other learner-related factors can potentially influence learning processes and outcomes: executive functions, working memory capacity, motivational variables, and interest. The conceptual model refers to individual learner characteristics in order to capture aptitude—treatment interactions (Snow, 1991), the expertise reversal effect (Kalyuga, 2007), and other motivational and affective predictors of learning outcomes with moderate to high effects (see Lazowski & Hulleman, 2016 for an overview). In line with research findings on the role of working memory (e.g., Koopmann-Holm & O'Connor, 2017; Sweller, 2005) and executive functions (Miyake & Friedman, 2012; Schwaighofer et al., 2015), we hypothesize that these factors might moderate both learning processes and outcomes.

2.2.3 Diagnostic Activities

Diagnostic processes require the collection, integration, and generation of case-specific information to reduce uncertainty and make medical or educational decisions. Therefore, we hypothesize that these processes require the same activities that are used across domains to collect and generate knowledge. The taxonomy of eight activities relevant to diagnostic processes was adopted from research on scientific reasoning and argumentation (Fischer et al., 2014). These activities include problem identification, questioning, hypothesis generation, construction/redesign of artifacts, evidence generation, evidence evaluation, drawing conclusions, and communicating the results. Diagnosing may require all or only some of these activities, the order of these activities may vary, with some activities repeated and some skipped depending on the particular situation at hand.

2.2.4 Diagnostic Quality: Accuracy and Efficiency

Diagnostic quality consists of the two measures diagnostic accuracy and diagnostic efficiency. Accuracy is a measure of the correspondence between the true state of the person being diagnosed and the diagnosis. In medical education, this would refer to correctly identifying the disease; in teacher education, this would relate to the assessment of the student's knowledge, their competence, or the identification of misconceptions. The second variable is diagnostic efficiency, which refers to the time, effort, and costs required to reach an accurate diagnosis and contributes to the quality of the diagnosis alongside diagnostic accuracy.

2.2.5 Simulations as Instructional Method

To develop professional competencies, learners need to have sufficient prior knowledge at their disposal and engage in a large amount of practice (i.e., Van Lehn, 1996). Simulations allow learners to practice authentic cases without compromising patients' or students' safety or well-being, and address rare and complex situations. Simulations also provide sufficient time and opportunity for practice, understanding underlying principles and concepts, and developing reasoning and reflection skills (Frasson & Blanchard, 2012).

2.2.6 Explicit Presentation of Information

Presenting information explicitly may play an important role in designing learning environments that facilitate the development of competences. Domain concepts and strategies, the framework of the task, and its requirements need to be communicated to guide students' attention to the most relevant information and reduce confusion (Kirschner et al., 2006; Sweller, 2005). However, there is no systematic research on how much explicit information needs to be communicated in different domains and learning environments. Moreover, research on the role of and interaction between the explicit presentation of information and other instructional methods is scarce. How the explicit presentation of information can be included in simulations is further described in Chaps. 6 and 7.

2.2.7 Scaffolding

The most prominent definition of scaffolding (Wood et al., 1976) defines it as the process of supporting learners by taking over some intricate factors of the task. According to recent literature reviews (Belland, 2014; Reiser & Tabak, 2014), scaffolding is effective in supporting the development of complex cognitive skills. It can facilitate cognitive, metacognitive, motivational and strategic learning processes and outcomes (Hannafin et al., 1999). Some promising forms of support in simulation-based learning that have shown positive effects in facilitating learning are providing examples, prompts, role-taking, and introducing reflection phases.

Prompts refer to information or guidance offered to learners during the learning process in order to improve its effectiveness (Berthold et al., 2007). Empirical evidence provides support for self-explanation prompts (Heitzmann et al., 2015, 2019), metacognitive prompts (Quintana et al., 2004), and collaboration scripts (Fischer et al., 2013; Vogel et al., 2017) as supports for learning. How prompts can be used successfully in simulations is described in Chaps 5, 6, and 8.

Role-taking can be considered a type of scaffolding when it reduces the full complexity of a situation by assigning learners a specific role with limited tasks or a limited perspective on the full task. A large body of empirical research suggests that complex skills can be acquired effectively in the agent role (i.e., teacher or doctor) (e.g., Cook, 2014). Scaffolding for role-taking is implemented in the simulations described in Chaps. 4, 5, 9, and 10.

The positive effects of reflection on learning were first proposed by Dewey (1933). Reflection can be induced through guided reflection phases and can take place before, during, or after an event. Different types of reflection (e.g., reflecting on reasoning or reflecting on the problem at hand) have been reported to efficiently foster the acquisition of diagnostic competences in medicine (Sandars, 2009) and teacher education (Beauchamp, 2015). Reflection phases were included in the simulations described in Chap. 9.

2.2.8 The Nature of the Diagnostic Situation

The nature of the diagnostic situation is defined by the set of specific features present in the specific situation in which the diagnosis takes place (Heitzmann et al., 2019). Heitzmann et al. suggest differentiating these features along two dimensions: (1) the source of information for the diagnosis, and (2) the necessity to collaborate with other professionals to reach the diagnosis. With regard to the first dimension, a distinction can be made between interaction-based and document-based diagnoses. In a diagnosis based on interaction, the information is gathered through interaction with another person (e.g., patient, student, their family members, etc.), (see simulations described in Chaps. 4, 5, 6, and 9); conversely, document-based diagnosis relies on information obtained in written or recorded form (see simulations described in Chaps. 5, 7, and 9). This distinction is highly relevant for practice, as different information sources might require different processing times as well as different types and amount of scaffolding. The second dimension ranges from individual diagnostic actions to a necessity to collaborate and communicate with other professionals during the diagnostic process. The processes involved in such collaboration and the factors relevant for diagnostic efficiency and accuracy during it have not been thoroughly researched in either the medical or teacher education fields. Simulations involving a collaborative context are described in Chaps. 7 and 10.

2.2.9 Domain

We focused on medical and teacher education as two domains that require accurate diagnoses before further professional action can be taken. Simulations in medical education are described in Chaps. 9 and 10. Simulations in teacher education are described in Chaps. 3, 4, 5, 6, 7, and 8. There are some similarities in diagnostic processes and thus also in diagnostic competences between these two domains. Therefore, we assume that interdisciplinary research and applications of simulation-based learning can provide insights for both fields.

The diagnostic process in medicine aims to determine the cause of a disease and the appropriate course of action for either further diagnosis or treatment (Charlin et al., 2000). The diagnostic process in teacher education aims to identify the gap between the present and the desired state of learners' competences and optimize the use of instructional methods to close this gap (Helmke et al., 2012). While the two fields differ, it is also obvious that these diagnostic processes share a key commonality, namely that diagnosing a patient's health status or a learner's understanding is a goal-oriented process of collecting and integrating case-specific information to reduce uncertainty in order to make medical or educational decisions (Heitzmann et al., 2019).

2.3 Evidence from a Meta-Analysis

Recently, we conducted a meta-analysis of 35 empirical studies building on the conceptual framework developed above to investigate the role of instruction, scaffolding, and contextual factors in facilitating the development of diagnostic competences in learners with different levels (low and high) of professional knowledge. As little empirical research was found on the effects of simulation-based learning on the development diagnostic competences, a broader search was conducted and studies of different types of instructional support were included in the analysis. We specifically focused on investigating the role of problem-solving as one of several problem-centered instructional approaches (Belland et al., 2017, p. 311).

The main aim of the meta-analysis was to estimate the overall effect of instructional support on the development of diagnostic competences in the domains of medical and teacher education and, more specifically, provide the missing evidence and synthesized results on the effects of different scaffolding types. We also included learning with examples as a scaffolding type (in addition to prompts, role-taking and reflection phases). Examples allow learners to retrace the steps of a solution (worked example) or observe a model displaying the problem-solving process (modeling example) before they solve problems independently (Renkl, 2014). Instructional support had a moderate positive effect on diagnostic competences, which is in line with previous research findings on fostering complex cognitive skills (Belland et al., 2017; Dochy et al., 2003). Problem-based learning as an instructional support facilitated the improvement of diagnostic competences in all learners, independently of their prior professional knowledge base. However, it is important to note that all interventions that applied a problem-based learning approach also implemented at least one other type of scaffolding or additional instruction.

One of the research questions in the meta-analysis specifically addressed the interaction between individual learners' prerequisites (i.e., prior knowledge base) and the effectiveness of a problem-solving approach and scaffolding procedures. The hypothesis behind this research question was that scaffolding measures vary in the degree of self-regulation required from learners. Thus, we assumed that providing example solutions and modeling desired behavior are more strongly guided forms of instruction requiring less self-regulation, as the learners do not face a problem to solve, but rather a solution. In contrast, reflection phases were considered to require high levels of self-regulation. Diagnostic competences were found to be facilitated effectively through problem-solving independent of learners' knowledge base. Although all types of scaffolding had positive effects on learning, scaffolding types providing high levels of guidance were more effective for less advanced learners, whereas scaffolding types relying on high levels of self-regulation were more effective for more advanced learners.

Moreover, the context was a significant moderator of improved diagnostic competences, with better learning associated with an interactive diagnostic situation. The domains of medical and teacher education were comparable in the effects of instructional support and scaffolding, but differed in terms of the prior professional knowledge base and therefore presumably in the design of effective learning environments to foster diagnostic competences.

2.4 Conclusions

This chapter addressed existing theoretical and empirical research on developing competences in higher education. It aimed at describing state-of-the-art research and developing a theoretical framework for using problem-solving (with and without simulations) to facilitate the development of diagnostic competences in medical and teacher education. Existing research suggests that instructional support that uses problem-solving to facilitate the development of complex cognitive skills and competences, and in particular diagnostic competences, has a moderate positive effect on learning outcomes (Chernikova et al., 2019). Meta-analytical studies, in turn, provide evidence of positive effects of simulations, as an example of a problem-solving approach, on learning in multiple domains.

The existing research suffers from a vast heterogeneity with respect to how researchers define diagnosing and diagnostic competences, which individual learners' prerequisites and processes they assume to be relevant for diagnosing and learning to diagnose, what instructional approaches should be used, and how the context (i.e., the nature of the diagnostic situation) can influence the effectiveness of learning. Nevertheless, simulations are promising means to measure and facilitate diagnostic competences.

Notably, both the literature review and the meta-analysis identified a range of empirical studies that used different simulations to facilitate skills related to diagnostic competences; however, it also became clear that empirical studies rarely provide detailed descriptions of the learning environments and simulations involved or the measures used to assess improved competences. This makes it difficult to draw conclusions about effects of specific learning activities and processes.

Moreover, hardly any study reused existing simulation-based learning environments, preferring to design new ones from scratch and match them to the study's particular needs. Such an approach contributes to high levels of heterogeneity that is difficult to explain as well as difficulties in summarizing the applied methods. This in turn leads to a lack of standardized instruments and measures that can be systematically used and adjusted if needed. However, such efforts are necessary to create foundations for high-quality, interdisciplinary, replicable empirical research and for better-designed learning environments to effectively facilitate the acquisition of diagnostic competences.

Acknowledgments The research presented in this chapter was funded by a grant from the Deutsche Forschungsgemeinschaft (DFG-FOR 2385) to Frank Fischer and Tina Seidel (FI 792/12-1).

References

Anderson, J. R. (1983). *Cognitive science series. The architecture of cognition*. Lawrence Erlbaum Associates, Inc..

Beauchamp, C. (2015). Reflection in teacher education: Issues emerging from a review of current literature. *Reflective Practice: International and Multidisciplinary Perspectives, 16*(1), 123–141. https://doi.org/10.1080/14623943.2014.982525

Belland, B. R. (2014). Scaffolding: Definition, current debates, and future directions. In J. M. Spector, M. D. Merrill, J. Elen, & M. J. Bishop (Eds.), *Handbook of research on educational communications and technology* (4th ed., pp. 505–518). Springer. https://doi.org/10.1007/978-1-4614-3185-5_39

Belland, B. R., Walker, A. E., Kim, N. J., & Lefler, M. (2017). Synthesizing results from empirical research on computer-based scaffolding in STEM education: A meta-analysis. *Review of Educational Research, 87*(2), 309–344. https://doi.org/10.3102/0034654316670999

Berthold, K., Nückles, M., & Renkl, A. (2007). Do learning protocols support learning strategies and outcomes? The role of cognitive and metacognitive prompts. *Learning and Instruction, 17*(5), 564–577. https://doi.org/10.1016/j.learninstruc.2007.09.007

Charlin, B., Tardif, J., & Boshuizen, H. P. A. (2000). Script and medical diagnostic knowledge: Theory and applications for clinical reasoning instruction and research. *Academic Medicine: Journal of the Association of American Medical Colleges, 75*(2), 182–190. PMID: 10693854

Chernikova, O., Heitzmann, N., Fink, M. C., Timothy, V., Seidel, T., & Fischer, F. (2019). Facilitating diagnostic competences in higher education - a meta-analysis in medical and teacher education. *Educational Psychology Review*, 1–40. https://doi.org/10.1007/s10648-019-09492-2

Cook, D. A. (2014). How much evidence does it take? A cumulative meta-analysis of outcomes of simulation-based education. *Medical Education, 48*(8), 750–760. https://doi.org/10.1111/medu.12473

Cook, D. A., Brydges, R., Hamstra, S. J., Zendejas, B., Szostek, J. H., Wang, A. T., . . . Hatala, R. (2012). Comparative effectiveness of technology-enhanced simulation versus other instructional methods: A systematic review and meta-analysis. *Simulation in Healthcare, 7*(5), 308–320. https://doi.org/10.1097/SIH.0b013e3182614f95

Cook, D. A., Hamstra, S. J., Brydges, R., Zendejas, B., Szostek, J. H., Wang, A. T., Erwin, P. J., & Hatala, R. (2013). Comparative effectiveness of instructional design features in simulation-based education: Systematic review and meta-analysis. *Medical Teacher, 35*(1), 867–898. https://doi.org/10.3109/0142159X.2012.714886

Dochy, F., Segers, M., van den Bossche, P., & Gijbels, D. (2003). Effects of problem-based learning: A meta-analysis. *Learning and Instruction, 13*(5), 533–568. https://doi.org/10.1016/S0959-4752(02)00025-7

Dewey, J. (1933). How we think. A restatement of the relation of reflective thinking to the educative process (revised ed.), Boston: D. C. Heath.

Fischer, F., Kollar, I., Stegmann, K., & Wecker, C. (2013). Toward a script theory of guidance in computer-supported collaborative learning. *Educational Psychologist, 48*(1), 56–66. https://doi.org/10.1080/00461520.2012.748005

Fischer, F., Kollar, I., Ufer, S., Sodian, B., Hussmann, H., Pekrun, R., et al. (2014). Scientific reasoning and argumentation: Advancing an interdisciplinary research agenda in education. *Frontline Learning Research, 2*(2), 28–45. https://doi.org/10.14786/flr.v2i2.96

Förtsch, C., Sommerhoff, D., Fischer, F., Fischer, M. R., Girwidz, R., Obersteiner, A., Reiss, K., Stürmer, K., Siebeck, M., Schmidmaier, R., Seidel, T., Ufer, S., Wecker, C., & Neuhaus, B. J. (2018). Systematizing professional knowledge of medical doctors and teachers: Development of an interdisciplinary framework in the context of diagnostic competences. *Education Sciences, 8*(4), 207. https://doi.org/10.3390/educsci8040207

Frasson, C., & Blanchard, E. (2012). Simulation-based learning. In I. N. Seel (Ed.), *Encyclopedia of the sciences of learning* (pp. 3076–3080). Springer.

Hannafin, M., Land, S., & Oliver, K. (1999). Open learning environments: Foundations, methods, and models. In C. M. Reigeluth (Ed.), *Instructional design theories and models: A new paradigm of instructional theory* (pp. 115–140). Lawrence Erlbaum Associates, Inc.

Heitzmann, N., Fischer, F., Kühne-Eversmann, L., & Fischer, M. R. (2015). Enhancing diagnostic competence with self-explanation prompts and adaptable feedback. *Medical Education, 49*(10), 993–1003. https://doi.org/10.1111/medu.12778

Heitzmann, N., Seidel, T., Opitz, A., Hetmanek, A., Wecker, C., Fischer, M., Ufer, S., Schmidmaier, R., Neuhaus, B., Siebeck, M., Stürmer, K., Obersteiner, A., Reiss, K., Girwidz, R., & Fischer, F. (2019). Facilitating diagnostic competences in simulations: A conceptual framework and a research agenda for medical and teacher education. *Frontline Learning Research, 7*(4), 1–24. https://doi.org/10.14786/flr.v7i4.384

Helmke, A., Schrader, F.-W., & Helmke, T. (2012). EMU: Evidenzbasierte Methoden der Unterrichtsdiagnostik und -entwicklung. Unterrichtsdiagnostik – Ein Weg, um Unterrichten sichtbar zu machen. *Schulverwaltung Bayern, 35*(6), 180–183.

Jonassen, D. H. (1997). Instructional design models for well-structured and ill-structured problem solving learning outcomes. *Educational Technology Research & Development, 45*(1), 45–94. https://doi.org/10.1007/BF02299613

Kalyuga, S. (2007). Expertise reversal effect and its implications for learner-tailored instruction. *Educational Psychology Review, 19*(4), 509–539.

Kirschner, P. A., Sweller, J., & Clark, R. E. (2006). Why minimal guidance during instruction does not work: An analysis of the failure of constructivist, discovery, problem-based, experiential, and inquiry-based teaching. *Educational Psychologist, 41*(2), 75–86. https://doi.org/10.1207/s15326985ep4102_1

Koopmann-Holm, B., & O'Connor, A. (2017). *Working memory*. CRC Press.

Koparan, T., & Yılmaz, G. (2015). The effect of simulation-based learning on prospective teachers' inference skills in teaching probability. *Universal Journal of Educational Research, 3*(11), 775–786. https://doi.org/10.13189/ujer.2015.031101

Lazonder, A. W., & Harmsten, R. (2016). Meta-analysis of inquiry-based learning: Effects of guidance. *Review of Educational Research, 86*(3), 681–718. https://doi.org/10.3102/0034654315627366

Lazowski, R. A., & Hulleman, C. S. (2016). Motivation interventions in education: A meta-analytic review. *Review of Educational Research, 86*(2), 602–640. https://doi.org/10.3102/0034654315617832

Liaw, S. Y., Chen, F. G., Klainin, P., Brammer, J., O'Brien, A., & Samarasekera, D. D. (2010). Developing clinical competency in crisis event management: An integrated simulation problem-based learning activity. *Advances in Health Sciences Education: Theory and Practice, 15*(3), 403–413. https://doi.org/10.1007/s10459-009-9208-9

Matsuda, N., Yarzebinski, E., Keiser, V., Raizada, R., Stylianides, G. J., & Koedinger, K. R. (2013). Studying the effect of a competitive game show in a learning by teaching environment. *International Journal of Artificial Intelligence in Education, 23*(1–4), 1–21. https://doi.org/10.1007/s40593-013-0009-1

Miyake, A., & Friedman, N. P. (2012). The nature and organization of individual differences in executive functions: Four general conclusions. *Current Directions in Psychological Science, 21*(1), 8–14. https://doi.org/10.1177/0963721411429458

Quintana, C., Reiser, B. J., Davis, E. A., Krajcik, J., Fretz, E., Duncan, R. G., Kyza, E., Edelson, D., & Soloway, E. (2004). A scaffolding design framework for software to support science inquiry. *Journal of the Learning Sciences, 13*(3), 337–386. https://doi.org/10.1207/s15327809jls1303_4

Reiser, B. J., & Tabak, I. (2014). Scaffolding. In R. K. Sawyer (Ed.), *Cambridge handbooks in psychology. The Cambridge handbook of the learning sciences* (pp. 44–62). Cambridge University Press. https://doi.org/10.1017/CBO9781139519526.005

Renkl, A. (2014). Toward an instructionally oriented theory of example-based learning. *Cognitive Science, 38*(1), 1–37. https://doi.org/10.1111/cogs.12086

Renkl, A., & Atkinson, R. K. (2003). Structuring the transition from example study to problem solving in cognitive skill acquisition: A cognitive load perspective. *Educational Psychologist, 38*(1), 15–22. https://doi.org/10.1207/S15326985EP3801_3

Sandars, J. (2009). The use of reflection in medical education: AMEE guide no. 44. *Medical Teacher, 31*(8), 685–695. https://doi.org/10.1080/01421590903050374

Schwaighofer, M., Fischer, F., & Bühner, M. (2015). Does working memory training transfer? A meta-analysis including training conditions as moderators. *Educational Psychologist, 50*(2), 138–166. https://doi.org/10.1080/00461520.2015.1036274

Seidel, T., Stürmer, K., Schäfer, S., & Jahn, G. (2015). How preservice teachers perform in teaching events regarding generic teaching and learning components. *Zeitschrift Für Entwicklungspsychologie Und Pädagogische Psychologie, 47*(2), 84–96. https://doi.org/10.1026/0049-8637/a000125

Shannon, R. E. (1975). *Systems simulation: The art and science*. Prentice-Hall.

Shavelson, R. J. (2013). On an approach to testing and modeling competence. *Educational Psychologist, 48*(2), 73–86. https://doi.org/10.1080/00461520.2013.779483

Shulman, L. S. (1987). Knowledge and teaching: Foundations of the new reform. *Harvard Educational Review, 57*(1), 1–23.

Snow, R. E. (1991). Aptitude-treatment interaction as a framework for research on individual differences in psychotherapy. *Journal of Consulting and Clinical Psychology, 59*(2), 205–210.

Stark, R., Kopp, V., & Fischer, M. R. (2011). Case-based learning with worked examples in complex domains: Two experimental studies in undergraduate medical education. *Learning and Instruction, 21*(1), 22–33. https://doi.org/10.1016/j.learninstruc.2009.10.001

Sweller, J. (2005). Implications of cognitive load theory for multimedia learning. In R. E. Mayer (Ed.), *The Cambridge handbook of multimedia learning* (pp. 19–30). Cambridge University Press.

Van Lehn, K. (1996). Cognitive skill acquisition. *Annual Review of Psychology, 47*(1), 513–539. https://doi.org/10.1146/annurev.psych.47.1.513

Vogel, F., Wecker, C., Kollar, I., & Fischer, F. (2017). Socio-cognitive scaffolding with computer-supported collaboration scripts: A meta-analysis. *Educational Psychology Review, 29*(3), 477–511. https://doi.org/10.1007/s10648-016-9361-7

Wissenschaftsrat. (2014). Bedeutung und Weiterentwicklung von simulation in der Wissenschaft [importance of the development of simulations in science].

Wood, D., Bruner, J. S., & Ross, G. (1976). The role of tutoring in problem solving. *Journal of Child Psychology and Psychiatry, 17*(2), 89–100. https://doi.org/10.1111/j.1469-7610.1976.tb00381.x

Open Access This chapter is licensed under the terms of the Creative Commons Attribution 4.0 International License (http://creativecommons.org/licenses/by/4.0/), which permits use, sharing, adaptation, distribution and reproduction in any medium or format, as long as you give appropriate credit to the original author(s) and the source, provide a link to the Creative Commons license and indicate if changes were made.

The images or other third party material in this chapter are included in the chapter's Creative Commons license, unless indicated otherwise in a credit line to the material. If material is not included in the chapter's Creative Commons license and your intended use is not permitted by statutory regulation or exceeds the permitted use, you will need to obtain permission directly from the copyright holder.

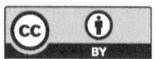

Chapter 3
Learning to Diagnose Primary Students' Mathematical Competence Levels and Misconceptions in Document-Based Simulations

Angelika Wildgans-Lang, Sarah Scheuerer, Andreas Obersteiner, Frank Fischer, and Kristina Reiss

This chapter's simulation at a glance

Domain	Teacher education
Topic	Diagnosing primary students' mathematical competence levels and misconceptions
Learner's task	To assume the role of a teacher and analyze students' documents to identify primary students' mathematical competence levels and misconceptions
Target group	Pre-service elementary teachers
Diagnostic mode	Document-based individual diagnosing
Sources of information	Primary students' solutions to mathematical tasks
Special features	All mathematical problems and students' solutions in the simulated environment come from pilot studies of VERA-3, a German large-scale comparison test in Grade 3, based on the primary level mathematical competence model by Reiss and Winkelmann (2009)

A. Wildgans-Lang (✉) · S. Scheuerer · A. Obersteiner · K. Reiss
Heinz Nixdorf Endowed Chair for Mathematics Education, TUM School of Social Sciences and Technology, Technical University of Munich (TUM), Munich, Germany
e-mail: a.wildgans-lang@tum.de

F. Fischer
Chair of Education and Educational Psychology, Department of Psychology, LMU Munich, Munich, Germany

© The Author(s) 2022
F. Fischer, A. Opitz (eds.), *Learning to Diagnose with Simulations*,
https://doi.org/10.1007/978-3-030-89147-3_3

3.1 Diagnosing as a Key for Adaptive Teaching

"Teachers need to be aware of what each and every student is thinking and knowing" (Hattie, 2010, p. 238). In addition to emphasizing the importance of teachers for students' learning progress in general, Hattie identifies as one of his signposts toward excellent education that teachers must be able to diagnose their students' current learning statuses in order to provide adequate and useful feedback (Hattie, 2010) and thus to teach adaptively. Such diagnostic competences can be defined as "individual dispositions enabling people to apply their knowledge in diagnostic activities according to professional standards to collect and interpret data in order to take decisions of high quality" (Heitzmann et al., 2019, p. 5). Diagnosing as a prerequisite for adaptive teaching has recently been studied by several research groups, including NeDiKo (e.g., Südkamp & Praetorius, 2017), DiaKom (Leuders et al., 2018) and Cosima (Chernikova et al., 2022; Heitzmann et al., 2019). Teachers' diagnostic competences have also received increased attention on the political level. In Germany, for instance, diagnosing has been included as a standard competence for adaptive teaching in the national teacher training standards (Standing Conference of the Ministers of Education and Cultural Affairs of the Länder in the Federal Republic of Germany—Kultusministerkonferenz, 2004b).

Despite its recognized relevance, diagnosing is not yet sufficiently taught during university teacher training. Oser and Oelkers (2001) point out that there is indeed a gap between the requirements of the teaching profession, especially with respect to diagnosing, and the content taught at university and during in-service teacher training. According to Shulman (1986), teachers should have a wide range of knowledge, including *content knowledge*, *pedagogical content knowledge* and *pedagogical knowledge*. Förtsch et al. (2018) illustrate the applicability of these categories to the context of diagnosing. In addition to the above categories of knowledge, Shulman further defined three "forms of knowledge" that describe how to *represent* these categories, namely *propositional knowledge, case knowledge,* and *strategic knowledge* (Shulman, 1986, p. 10). Propositional knowledge comprises theoretical foundations, formulated as "principles, maxims, and norms" (Shulman, 1986, p. 11). In contrast, *case knowledge* is "knowledge of specific, well-documented, and richly described events" and comprises "examples of specific instances of practice" (Shulman, 1986, p. 11). Accordingly, *case knowledge* helps to apply theoretical content about diagnosing in specific situations, such as diagnosing students' misconceptions in mathematics. Strategic knowledge is used in situations when "principles collide and no simple solution is possible" (Shulman, 1986, p. 11). However, in the everyday life of a teacher, classroom situations and in particular interactions with students may not simply be able to be abstracted to a general case, but may require adaptation to the individual circumstances. These circumstances probably also affect teachers' diagnostic judgments about their students. In summary, possessing knowledge in all three categories as well as all three forms may be beneficial for the teaching profession in general. Thus, supporting these various knowledge facets during teacher education may have a positive impact on prospective teachers' diagnostic processes and results. It is worth mentioning, however, that in addition to knowledge, diagnostic competences also include diagnostic activities (see Chernikova et al., 2022).

3.2 Learning from Other Disciplines About Supporting Diagnostic Processes in Simulated Learning Environments

Research on diagnosing in education has focused more strongly on the outcome of diagnosing rather than on the diagnostic process (Artelt & Rausch, 2014). Medical research on diagnosing has, however, more intensively studied diagnostic processes (see Fink et al., 2022; Radkowitsch et al., 2022). In our research, we adopt a general framework to analyze the diagnostic processes with respect to epistemic-diagnostic activities (Fischer et al., 2014), hereafter referred to as diagnostic activities. In particular, we aim to assess which diagnostic activities occur during diagnosing in educational settings, to measure their frequency and their influence on diagnostic results.

In a first practice trial (Wildgans-Lang et al., 2019), we found that we can apply the model of diagnostic activities (Fischer et al., 2014) in the educational setting under study. More specifically, we found that teachers identify problems in mathematics on the basis of questions, incorrect student solutions, or student mistakes on homework and tests. In some cases, teachers ask themselves which misconceptions can occur in a specific topic area before the lesson starts and formulate hypotheses accordingly. If teachers then create specific tasks to identify such misconceptions, this is referred to as *artifact construction*; if teachers select from a set of existing tasks, this is called *evidence generation*. These diagnostic activities can already occur during lesson preparation. Further diagnostic activities are *evidence evaluation*, which involves recognizing a mistake in the student's solution, *evaluating* it by applying their pedagogical content knowledge, and drawing appropriate *conclusions* to communicate to the student, class, parents, or colleagues (Fischer et al., 2014).

The Nediko group has developed a model in which the diagnostic activities and their sequence are discussed. The group describes that—if the diagnostic result is not obvious—the generation of hypotheses is necessary. For this, information about the student's mathematical competences must be collected (evidence generation and evaluation) and then evaluated; that is, conclusions must be drawn, which can lead to further hypotheses (Herppich et al., 2017). The three-step diagnostic process in "error situations" (Heinrichs & Kaiser, 2018, p. 79) also refers to diagnostic activities (Heinrichs, 2015; Heinrichs & Kaiser, 2018). In summary, central to all these diagnostic processes is the generation of hypotheses, which is based on evidence generation and evaluation and from which conclusions are drawn.

3.3 Diagnosing Based on Students' Solutions

Teachers often diagnose students' competences or misconceptions when they identify an error in students' work (Wildgans-Lang et al., 2019) or with the aim to evaluate their performance. Often the focus is on ranking students' performance (Artelt & Rausch, 2014). However, a more important indicator would be to evaluate students' competences with regard to clearly defined standards, such as the mathematical competence levels model for the primary level (Reiss & Winkelmann, 2009). This model divides the mathematical competences acquired by German primary school students in their first four school years into five levels. These range from basic technical knowledge (via routine procedures) (Level 1) to modeling complex problems and independently finding appropriate strategies (Level 5; see Reiss & Obersteiner, 2019). In addition, the competences are divided into domains, such as numbers and operations or patterns and structures, hereafter referred to as competence areas, which are in turn based on guiding principles of the national curriculum (Kultusministerkonferenz, 2004a). This theoretical classification of competences to be acquired in primary school has been reviewed in recent years via comparative studies throughout Germany (Stanat, 2012). Students' misconceptions can also be classified into these competence areas. Misconceptions are often the reason for systematic errors (Radatz, 1980). In the first 4 years of school, students learn many basic skills in mathematics. Typical mistakes regarding such basic skills include, for example, misconceptions about place value. Such misconceptions may lead to errors when adding two numbers digit by digit. Descriptions of typical errors and misconceptions can be found in Padberg and Benz (2011). Typical errors in the modeling process encompass errors in understanding word problems, developing a solution plan, omitting steps when solving the problem, and correctly interpreting the result (Franke et al., 2010).

3.4 Supporting Diagnosing in a Simulated Environment

A simulated learning environment to support diagnosing may enhance the user's content knowledge, pedagogical content knowledge, and pedagogical knowledge about diagnosing. Furthermore, it should give the user the opportunity to apply their knowledge about diagnosing to authentic cases. Additionally, work in the learning environment can be stopped and repeated, which seems to be helpful for reflecting on the evidence and diagnostic activities already carried out (Blomberg et al., 2013; Rich & Hannafin, 2009; Santagata, 2005). To support the transfer of the practiced diagnostic activities to real classroom situations, it might be beneficial for the learning environment to be as authentic as possible (Stammen et al., 2018).

3.5 Development of the Simulated Environment

In this section, we explain how we developed the learning environment based on the goals presented in the previous section. In order to convey *case knowledge* in the simulated learning environment, we developed appropriate *cases*. The main idea was to employ theory-driven design to generate documents depicting virtual students' solutions to mathematical problems. Based on these documents, the users of the learning environment had to diagnose the virtual students' mathematical competences.

The mathematical competence model on the primary level by Reiss and Winkelmann (2009) introduced above served as a foundation for developing the virtual students within the learning environment. In order to apply the model, we decided to generate virtual *third graders,* as students in this grade are already familiar with most of the mathematical content taught in elementary school. The virtual students were designed to have varying levels of mathematical knowledge, which in turn determined whether they would solve a given mathematical problem correctly or not. Their knowledge levels would also determine whether they made various types of mistakes when solving the problems.

All mathematical problems in the simulated environment were taken from pilot studies of VERA-3, a German large-scale comparison test for Grade 3 of elementary school. All VERA-3 problems included in the learning environment have undergone a thorough development process and are Rasch-scaled and empirically validated. The problems were developed based on the model of mathematical competence, such that each mathematical problem can be assigned to exactly one of the competence levels in the model. In other words, the competence model clearly and precisely describes which competence level is minimally necessary to solve a specific mathematical problem correctly. Furthermore, each mathematical problem is assigned to a single content area in line with curricular standards.

For simplicity's sake, we restricted the content of the mathematical problems to two competence areas: *numbers and operations* and *patterns and structures* (see Reiss & Obersteiner, 2019; Reiss & Winkelmann, 2009). *Numbers and operations* comprise arithmetic problems on the primary level. Due to its central role in primary mathematics education and its fundamental importance for other competence areas (Rasch & Schütte, 2007), *numbers and operations* is a well-researched competence area, particularly with respect to typical student mistakes and error strategies. The competence area *patterns and structures*—which primarily requires recognizing connections and contexts related to the given information in mathematical problems—is also fundamentally related to other competence areas and therefore relevant to a wide range of mathematical content (Wittmann & Müller, 2007). Thus, due to their close relations to other competence areas, the competence areas *numbers and operations* as well as *patterns and structures* seem to be suitable as a starting point for developing the learning environment. Figs. 3.1 and 3.2 show mathematical problems in the two competence areas.

> Write the numbers in ascending order.
> 315, 887, 88, 1002, 351
>
> ____ < ____ < ____ < ____ < ____

Fig. 3.1 Sample problem for the competence area numbers and operations. The text was translated from the German original by the authors. (Further examples: https://www.iqb.hu-berlin.de/vera/aufgaben/map)

> One pencil costs 1 euro in a shop.
> For 10 pencils you have to pay 9 euro.
>
> Fill in the cheapest price for 7, 13 and 20 pencils.
>
> | Number of pencils | 7 | 13 | 20 |
> |---|---|---|---|
> | Price | ___ | ___ | ___ |

Fig. 3.2 Sample problem for the competence area patterns and structures. The text was translated from the German original by the authors. (Further examples: https://www.iqb.hu-berlin.de/vera/aufgaben/map)

We carefully selected mathematical problems for the learning environment from 50,000 original student solutions by participants in VERA-3 pilot studies from 2015 to 2017. A "student solution" is a student's response to a single mathematical problem. This means that the 50,000 student solutions include both responses by *different students* to the *same problem* and responses by the *same student* to *different problems*. The student solutions concerned problems assigned to the two competence areas discussed before. The problem selection process involved three steps:

- In the first step, we theoretically described typical misconceptions by primary students in the two competence areas based on Padberg and Benz (2011) as well as Franke et al. (2010). We decided to focus on two facets of misconceptions: misconceptions in arithmetic (such as misconceptions concerning the place value system or the number zero) and misconceptions with regard to word problems (such as misconceptions concerning verbal answers to word problems).
- In the second step, we studied the original student solutions from VERA-3 to identify mistakes attributable to the misconceptions defined in the first step. We grouped student solutions with mistakes stemming from the same misconception.
- In the third step, we compared these groups of student solutions (each representing one misconception), paying particular regard to two further aspects. First, we wanted to keep the number of mathematical problems in the learning environment limited. For this reason, we preferred problems with student solutions assigned to several misconceptions. In other words, we excluded problems

that did not result in mistakes regarding different competence areas and misconceptions. Second, we sought to select student solutions with similar handwriting in order to make the simulated environment as authentic as possible. As a result, we removed solutions with particularly conspicuous or unique handwriting.

After these steps, a set of 55 mathematical problems uniquely assigned to one of the five levels in the competence model were selected. For each of the 55 problems, we collected up to 15 original student solutions. In total, this resulted in 520 student solutions.

Finally, we developed virtual students with varying levels of mathematical competence. We assigned each virtual student a particular misconception determined beforehand. For simplicity's sake, each virtual student exhibited only one misconception. Based on the groups of student solutions identified in the second step, we assigned each virtual student original VERA-3 solutions with mistakes reflecting the corresponding misconception. We also assigned each virtual student correctly solved VERA-3 solutions based on the student's competence level.

Note that we considered the empirical solution rates from VERA for each competence level when assigning the problems and corresponding solutions to the virtual students. More precisely, we ensured that a virtual student on a particular competence level would solve at least half of the mathematical problems on this competence level correctly. Accordingly, each student solved considerably fewer problems correctly on higher competence levels, because the requirements of these problems exceed the student's mathematical abilities. By contrast, the student solved most problems that are assigned to a lower competence level correctly.

In total, we developed 15 virtual students with different misconceptions, each of which was assigned different original VERA-3 solutions. The selected mathematical problems covered all five levels of the mathematical competence model. On the basis of their individual misconceptions and mathematical competences, the virtual students were distributed across the levels of the competence level model as follows:

- four virtual students had Competence Level 1,
- three virtual students had Competence Level 2,
- four virtual students had Competence Level 3,
- two virtual students had Competence Level 4, and
- two virtual students had Competence Level 5.

Compared to the results of a standardization study in Germany, students on Competence Level 1 are somewhat over-represented in the simulated environment. This is due to the fact that students with the fundamental misconceptions we considered important are often at Competence Level 1.

We also assigned names to the virtual students. We selected short and common names from a list of the most popular names for newborns in Germany in 2011. This year corresponds approximately to the birth year of the virtual third graders at the time the simulated environment was developed. The virtual students' gender was

Table 3.1 Overview of the competence levels, students and their misconceptions

Competence level	Student	Misconception concerning...
1	1	Place value system (Padberg & Benz, 2011, 108, 123)
	2	Modeling task misconception (compare e.g., Franke et al., 2010, pp. 114–115)
	3	Switching between different representations (Hasemann & Gasteiger, 2014, pp. 109–118)
	4	Multiplication and division (Padberg & Benz, 2011, 148, 167–168)
2	5	Reading text-intensive word problems
	6	Column addition (Padberg & Benz, 2011, pp. 229–231)
	7	Calculations with the number zero (Padberg & Benz, 2011, 147–148, 167)
3	8	Completeness of the solution to word problems (Franke et al., 2010, pp. 114–115)
	9	Place value system (advanced)
	10	Formulation of verbal answers (Franke et al., 2010, pp. 114–115)
	11	Structured approach when solving word problems (Franke et al., 2010, pp. 114–115)
4	12	Symbolism and terminology
	13	Completeness of the solution to word problems (advanced) (Franke et al., 2010, pp. 114–115)
5	14	Formulation of verbal answers (advanced) (Franke et al., 2010, pp. 114–115)
	15	No misconception

roughly equally distributed. Table 3.1 provides an overview of the 15 virtual students developed and their corresponding misconceptions.

3.6 Operating Principle of the Environment

Upon entering the simulated learning environment, users (in our case pre-service elementary teachers) first complete a knowledge test. This test assesses Shulman's three types of knowledge (content knowledge, pedagogical knowledge, and pedagogical content knowledge; see Shulman, 1986). The test was included to be able to analyze the relations between teachers' knowledge base and their diagnostic process and results.

After finishing the knowledge test, users are introduced to the learning setting. They are asked to imagine they are the teacher of a third-grade class and need to diagnose their students' mathematical learning statuses. This means assigning the students to one of the five levels of the competence model, which is briefly introduced at the beginning as well. They are also asked to identify the students' mathematical misconceptions. Users (pre-service teachers) are told that they will

3 Learning to Diagnose Primary Students' Mathematical Competence Levels... 25

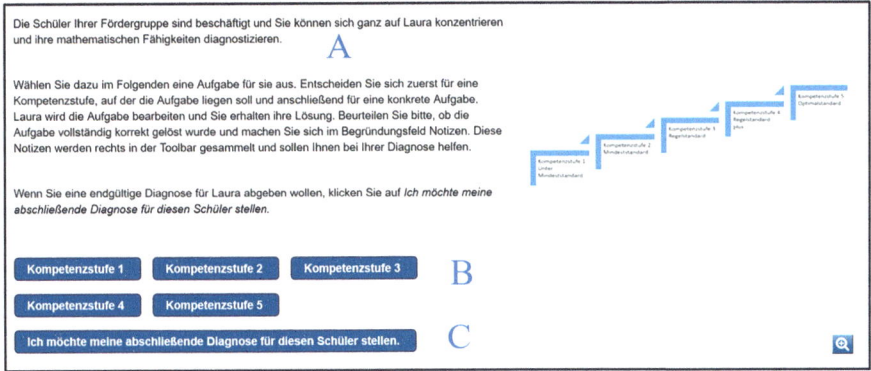

Fig. 3.3 Screenshot of the learning environment including instructions (A), buttons with competence levels (B) and a button for making the final diagnosis (C). The right side of the screen shows the five competence levels in the model

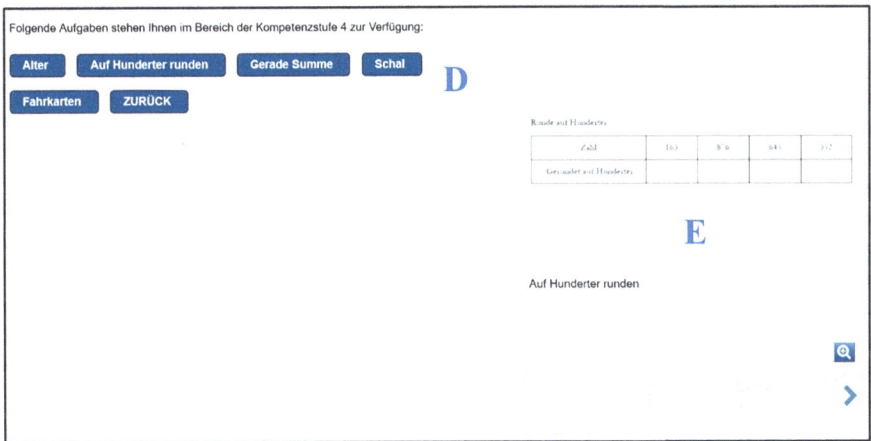

Fig. 3.4 Screenshot of the learning environment showing the titles of the available mathematical problems (D) and one problem preview (E) for one virtual student

communicate individually with each student while all other students in the class work quietly at their desks (see also Fig. 3.3, letter A).

During the diagnostic process, pre-service teachers first choose which one of the 15 virtual students in the simulated environment they want to diagnose by analyzing his or her solutions to mathematical problems. The available problems for the selected student are sorted by difficulty according to the five competence levels (see Fig. 3.3, letter B). The pre-service teachers first select a competence level (see Fig. 3.3, letter B) and subsequently are presented with titles (see Fig. 3.4, letter D) as well as previews (see Fig. 3.4, letter E) of the available mathematical problems for the selected student on the selected competence level. For each of the 15 virtual

Runde auf Hunderter.				
Zahl	163	876	645	352
Gerundet auf Hunderter	37	24	55	48

Fig. 3.5 One virtual student's solution to a mathematical problem on Competence Level 4. The student has been asked to round to the nearest multiple of 100

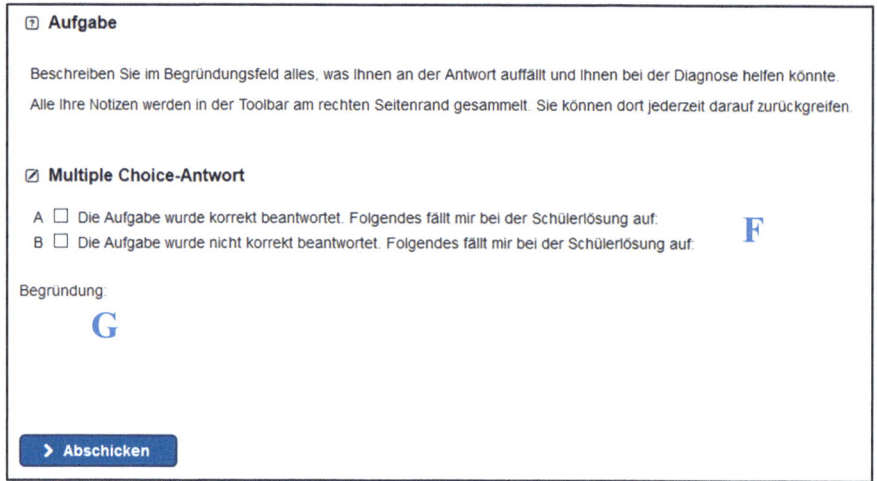

Fig. 3.6 Screenshot of the learning environment where the user is asked to judge the correctness of the student solution (F) and to take notes (G)

students, between five and eight mathematical problems are available for each competence level. Evidence generation in this learning environment means that the pre-service teacher decides which problem to select and then clicks the appropriate button. The student's solution to the mathematical problem appears right away (see Fig. 3.5). The teachers are asked to judge the correctness of the student solution (see Fig. 3.6, letter F) and to take notes (see Fig. 3.6, letter G) that may help to diagnose the student's mathematical learning status. In this way, pre-service teachers can examine the student's solutions to various problems and take notes until they think they have collected enough information to make a final diagnosis. The notes taken can be viewed throughout the entire process. On the one hand, the notes serve as a recall aid for teachers when they make their final diagnosis. On the other hand, we expect that these notes could provide insights into the diagnostic process. For example, it will be interesting to see whether the pre-service teachers mainly write down observations or whether they also hypothesize and draw conclusions, and how these diagnostic activities are related to the diagnostic results. A challenge will be to code the notes such that they can be assigned to different diagnostic activities (Fischer et al., 2014).

At any point, the pre-service teachers can elect to make a final diagnosis (see Fig. 3.3, letter C), which comprises several steps: First, the teachers have to choose and justify the student's competence level and estimate the certainty of their decision on a scale from 0% to 100%. Then, the teachers have to describe the virtual student's misconception in a free-text entry. After that, the teachers are supposed to select the student's misconception out of a set of five misconceptions provided. Here again, the teachers are asked to rate the certainty of their decision on a scale from 0% to 100%. By asking for the certainty of the teachers' decisions, we aim to distinguish between well-reasoned decisions and guessing. Furthermore, we want to analyze whether decisions are better justified and precise after having diagnosed several students. Finally, after making a final diagnosis for this virtual student, the teacher can continue on to diagnosing the mathematical learning status of another student.

3.7 Preliminary Findings

In a first pilot study, the simulated environment was tested with 91 participants (77 female, 14 male, M = 22.9 years old, SD = 2.96, range 20–39 years old) from two universities in Germany. They were pre-service elementary school teachers in their first to ninth semester of university teacher education studies (M = 3.6). The pre-service teachers described the simulated environment and in particular the virtual children as authentic and motivating (Wildgans-Lang et al., 2020).

First data analyses show great variation in the pre-service elementary teachers' diagnostic processes. For instance, some participants selected a mathematical problem on Competence Level 3 to start. Depending on the student's solution to these problems, they continued with problems with a lower or higher level of difficulty. In contrast, some pre-service teachers consistently started the diagnostic process by selecting a mathematical problem on either Competence Level 1 or 5. These participants then selected problems with an increasing or decreasing level of difficulty, respectively, until they reached a decision. Our participants' diagnostic processes also greatly varied in the number of instances of evidence generation utilized (i.e., the number of mathematical problems used to diagnose one student). The number of problems used did not correlate with the accuracy of the diagnostic results, suggesting that viewing more evidence is not per se a good predictor of accurate diagnosing. It is also noteworthy that our participants rarely generated hypotheses, which we consider important in the diagnostic process. For a more detailed report on the results of this pilot study, see Wildgans-Lang et al. (2020).

After the pre-service teachers finished working with the learning environment, we asked them to describe in a short text how they proceeded when diagnosing their students, in particular, how they selected appropriate problems for the students and whether they found the allocation of problems to competence levels helpful. With this task, we wanted the teachers to reflect on their diagnostic process once more. In addition, we expected to identify aspects that were particularly important to teachers but that might not be recognizable from the data alone.

In general, most pre-service teachers reported that the classification of mathematical problems into competence levels was useful. One participant, for instance, reported that she began diagnosing by providing the students with problems on Level 2 in order to avoid challenging them too much at the beginning. Subsequently, this participant reported choosing problems that covered a similar mathematical topic as the previous problem, but on a higher competence level. After that, this participant selected other topics on the higher competence level. Another participant reported: "I always started with problems on Competence Level 1 and considered three student solutions. When I felt that the student solved the problems well and without mistakes, I continued with problems on the next (higher) competence level" (translated). Here again, the allocation of problems into competence levels seemed to be helpful.

However, a few participants indicated that working with the competence levels was more of a hindrance than helpful. They argued that their focus was on students' misconceptions. Therefore, they did not select problems based on the competence level but rather on the mathematical content. Hence, sorting the problems by level of difficulty was not helpful for these participants.

This feedback suggests that the majority of prospective teachers in our study focused more strongly on diagnosing students' competence levels rather than diagnosing their specific misconceptions. In fact, our participants diagnosed the students' competence level correctly in 75% of cases, while they diagnosed the correct misconception in less than one-third of cases (Wildgans-Lang et al., 2020).

3.8 Conclusion, Discussion, and Outlook

Apart from the data generated while teachers make a final diagnosis concerning a student's mathematical learning status (i.e., choosing his or her competence level and misconception), the simulated environment also records various data generated during the diagnostic process. Examples are the mathematical problems selected and their corresponding competence levels. Analyzing these data may help us understand (prospective) teachers' approaches to diagnosing students' mathematical learning status and compare these different approaches with the corresponding diagnostic results. Whether some approaches lead to better diagnostic results than others is an interesting question for further research. Moreover, analyzing the notes taken by teachers in the learning environment will be of particular interest for better understanding diagnostic processes. Specifically, we will categorize teachers' notes based on the aforementioned theoretical taxonomy of diagnostic activities. This categorization is intended to make the diagnostic process more tangible. Another question for further research is whether diagnostic processes and results depend on pre-service teachers' previous knowledge, such as that acquired during in-service teaching experiences or university courses, for example.

In summary, contributing to the first four overarching research questions mentioned in the introduction by Fischer et al. (2022) and in the concluding chapter by Opitz et al. (2022), the overarching goal for our future research will be to explore which circumstances and activities in the diagnostic process facilitate accurate diagnostic results. Identifying such factors will help us refine the simulated environment to more effectively foster pre-service teachers' diagnostic competences. Fostering diagnostic competences includes but is not limited to effectively conveying essential categories and forms of knowledge about diagnosing (see Shulman, 1986; Förtsch et al., 2018). The learning environment we have constructed for pre-service teachers should also serve as a platform to practice diagnosing and prepare for their future careers as teachers.

As one instructional approach, we are planning on implementing scaffolds in the learning environment. The idea of scaffolds is to provide minimal and targeted support to guide the learner to engage in well-thought-out diagnostic processes leading to accurate results. Such scaffolds could be strategic tips on how to carry out diagnostic activities. Scaffolds might be also content-related, providing tips concerning the mathematical competence model or common misconceptions among elementary students.

More generally, we aim to develop a simulated environment that has been empirically found to effectively support pre-service teachers' diagnostic competences when deployed as part of university teacher education. Such a learning environment will certainly not replace existing courses or real-life internships in schools, but may be used to complement them. Of course, how to optimally integrate such simulations into teacher education is a research question in its own right.

Acknowledgments The research presented in this chapter was funded by a grant from the Deutsche Forschungsgemeinschaft (DFG-FOR 2385) to Kristina Reiss, Andreas Obersteiner, and Frank Fischer (RE 1247/12-1; OB 412/3-1).

References

Artelt, C., & Rausch, T. (2014). Accuracy of teacher judgments. In S. Krolak-Schwerdt, S. Glock, & M. Böhmer (Eds.), *Teachers' professional development: Assessment, training, and learning* (The future of education research) (Vol. 03, pp. 27–43). Sense Publishers.

Blomberg, G., Renkl, A., Gamoran Sherin, M., Borko, H., & Seidel, T. (2013). Five research-based heuristics for using video in pre-service teacher education. *Journal for Educational Research Online / Journal für Bildungsforschung Online, 5*(1), 90–114.

Chernikova, O., Heitzmann, N., Opitz, A., Seidel, T., & Fischer, F. (2022). A theoretical framework for fostering diagnostic competences with simulations. In F. Fischer & A. Opitz (Eds.), *Learning to diagnose with simulations - examples from teacher education and medical education*. Springer.

Fink, M., Siebeck, M., Fischer, F., & Fischer, M. (2022). Live and video simulations of medical history taking: Theoretical background, design, development and validation of a learning environment. In F. Fischer & A. Opitz (Eds.), *Learning to diagnose with simulations - examples from teacher education and medical education*. Springer.

Fischer, F., Kollar, I., Ufer, S., Sodian, B., Hussmann, H., Pekrun, R., et al. (2014). Scientific reasoning and argumentation: Advancing an interdisciplinary research agenda in education. *Frontline Learning Research, 2*, 28–45. https://doi.org/10.14786/flr.v2i2.96

Fischer, F., Chernikova, O., & Opitz, A. (2022). Learning to diagnose with simulations: Introduction. In F. Fischer & A. Opitz (Eds.). *Learning to diagnose with simulations – examples from teacher education and medical education.* Springer.

Förtsch, C., Sommerhoff, D., Fischer, F., Fischer, M., Girwidz, R., Obersteiner, A., et al. (2018). Systematizing professional knowledge of medical doctors and teachers: Development of an interdisciplinary framework in the context of diagnostic competences. *Education Sciences, 8*, 207. https://doi.org/10.3390/educsci8040207

Franke, M., Padberg, F., & Ruwisch, S. (2010). *Didaktik des Sachrechnens in der Grundschule.* Spektrum Akademischer Verlag.

Hasemann, K., & Gasteiger, H. (2014). Mathematik Primarstufe und Sekundarstufe I + II. In *Anfangsunterricht Mathematik* (3rd ed.). Springer Spektrum.

Hattie, J. (2010). *Visible learning: A synthesis of over 800 meta-analyses relating to achievement.* Routledge.

Heinrichs, H. (2015). *Diagnostische Kompetenz von Mathematik-Lehramtsstudierenden: Messung und Förderung (Perspektiven der Mathematikdidaktik).* Springer Spektrum.

Heinrichs, H., & Kaiser, G. (2018). Diagnostic competence for dealing with students' errors: Fostering diagnostic competence in error situations. In T. Leuders, K. Philipp, & J. Leuders (Eds.), *Diagnostic competence of mathematics teachers: Unpacking a complex construct in teacher education and teacher practice* (Mathematics teacher education) (Vol. 11, pp. 79–94). Springer International Publishing.

Heitzmann, N., Seidel, T., Opitz, A., Hetmanek, A., Wecker, C., Fischer, M., Ufer, S., Schmidmaier, R., Neuhaus, B., Siebeck, M., Stürmer, K., Obersteiner, A., Reiss, K., Girwidz, R., & Fischer, F. (2019). Facilitating diagnostic competences in simulations in higher education. *Frontline Learning Research, 7*(4), 1–24. https://doi.org/10.14786/flr.v7i4.384

Herppich, S., Praetorius, A.-K., Hetmanek, A., Glogger-Frey, I., Ufer, S., Leutner, D., et al. (2017). Ein Arbeitsmodell für die empirische Erforschung der diagnostischen Kompetenz von Lehrkräften. In A. Südkamp & A.-K. Praetorius (Eds.), *Diagnostische Kompetenz von Lehrkräften: Theoretische und methodische Weiterentwicklungen* (Pädagogische Psychologie und Entwicklungspsychologie) (Vol. 94, pp. 75–94). Waxmann Verlag GmbH.

Kultusministerkonferenz. (2004a). Bildungsstandards im Fach Mathematik für den Primarbereich: Beschluss vom 15.10.2004.

Kultusministerkonferenz. (2004b). Standards für die Lehrerbildung: Bildungswissenschaften. Beschluss der KMK vom 16.12.2004. Standing conference of the ministers of education and cultural Affairs of the Länder in the Federal Republic of Germany. http://www.kmk.org/fileadmin/Dateien/veroeffentlichungen_beschluesse/2004/2004_12_16-Standards-Lehrerbildung.pdf

Leuders, T., Philipp, K., & Leuders, J. (2018). *Diagnostic competence of mathematics teachers: Unpacking a complex construct in teacher education and teacher practice* (Mathematics teacher education) (Vol. 11). Springer International Publishing.

Oser, F., & Oelkers, J. (Eds.). (2001). *Die Wirksamkeit der Lehrerbildungssysteme: Von der Allrounderbildung zur Ausbildung professioneller Standards (Nationales Forschungsprogramm 33 - Wirksamkeit unserer Bildungssysteme).* Rüegger.

Padberg, F., & Benz, C. (2011). Mathematik Primar- und Sekundarstufe I + II: Didaktik der Mathematik. In *Didaktik der Arithmetik: Für Lehrerausbildung und Lehrerfortbildung* (4th ed.). Spektrum Akademischer Verlag.

Radatz, H. (1980). *Fehleranalysen im Mathematikunterricht.* Vieweg+Teubner Verlag.

Radkowitsch, A., Sailer, M., Fischer, M., Schmidmaier, R., & Fischer, F. (2022). Diagnosing collaboratively: A theoretical model and a simulation-based learning environment. In F. Fischer & A. Opitz (Eds.), *Learning to diagnose with simulations - examples from teacher education and medical education.* Springer.

Rasch, R., & Schütte, S. (2007). Zahlen und Operationen. In G. Walther (Ed.), *Bildungsstandards für die Grundschule: Mathematik konkret: [Aufgabenbeispiele, Unterrichtsanregungen, Fortbildungsideen]; mit CD-ROM* (2nd ed., pp. 66–88). Lehrer-Bücherei.

Reiss, K., & Obersteiner, A. (2019). Competence models as a basis for defining, understanding, and diagnosing students' mathematical competences. In A. Fritz, V. G. Haase, & P. Räsänen (Eds.), *The international handbook of math learning difficulties: From the laboratory to the classroom.* Springer.

Reiss, K., & Winkelmann, H. (2009). Kompetenzstufenmodelle für das Fach Mathematik im Primarbereich. In D. Granzer (Ed.), *Bildungsstandards Deutsch und Mathematik: [Leistungsmessung in der Grundschule]* (pp. 120–141). Beltz-Pädagogik.

Rich, P. J., & Hannafin, M. (2009). Video annotation tools: Technologies to scaffold, structure, and transform teacher reflection. *Journal of Teacher Education, 60*(1), 52–67.

Santagata, R. (2005). Practices and beliefs in mistake-handling activities: A video study of Italian and US mathematics lessons. *Teaching and Teacher Education, 21*, 491–508. https://doi.org/10.1016/j.tate.2005.03.004

Shulman, L. S. (1986). Those who understand: Knowledge growth in teaching. *Educational Researcher, 15*, 4–14. https://doi.org/10.3102/0013189X015002004

Stammen, A., Malone, K., & Irving, K. (2018). Effects of modeling instruction professional development on biology teachers' scientific reasoning skills. *Education Sciences, 8*, 119–138. https://doi.org/10.3390/educsci8030119

Stanat, P. (Ed.). (2012). *Kompetenzen von Schülerinnen und Schülern am Ende der vierten Jahrgangsstufe in den Fächern Deutsch und Mathematik: Ergebnisse des IQB-Ländervergleichs 2011.* Waxmann Verlag GmbH.

Südkamp, A., & Praetorius, A.-K. (2017). Diagnostische Kompetenz von Lehrkräften: Theoretische und methodische Weiterentwicklungen. In *Pädagogische Psychologie und Entwicklungspsychologie* (Vol. 94). Waxmann Verlag GmbH.

Wildgans-Lang, A., Obersteiner, A., & Reiss, K. (2019). Epistemisch-diagnostische Aktivitäten im Diagnoseprozess bei Lehrkräften im Mathematikunterricht. In T. Ehmke, P. Kuhl, & M. Pietsch (Eds.), *Lehrer. Bildung. Gestalten.: Beiträge zur empirischen Forschung in der Lehrerbildung* (pp. 281–291). Juventa Verlag GmbH.

Wildgans-Lang, A., Scheuerer, S., Obersteiner, A., Fischer, F., & Reiss, K. (2020). Analyzing prospective mathematics teachers' diagnostic processes in a simulated environment. *ZDM, 52*(2), 241–254.

Wittmann, E. C., & Müller, G. N. (2007). Muster und Strukturen als fachliches Konzept. In G. Walther (Ed.), *Bildungsstandards für die Grundschule: Mathematik konkret: [Aufgabenbeispiele, Unterrichtsanregungen, Fortbildungsideen]; mit CD-ROM* (2nd ed., pp. 42–65). Cornelsen Scriptor.

Open Access This chapter is licensed under the terms of the Creative Commons Attribution 4.0 International License (http://creativecommons.org/licenses/by/4.0/), which permits use, sharing, adaptation, distribution and reproduction in any medium or format, as long as you give appropriate credit to the original author(s) and the source, provide a link to the Creative Commons license and indicate if changes were made.

The images or other third party material in this chapter are included in the chapter's Creative Commons license, unless indicated otherwise in a credit line to the material. If material is not included in the chapter's Creative Commons license and your intended use is not permitted by statutory regulation or exceeds the permitted use, you will need to obtain permission directly from the copyright holder.

Chapter 4
Diagnosing Mathematical Argumentation Skills: A Video-Based Simulation for Pre-Service Teachers

Elias Codreanu, Sina Huber, Sarah Reinhold, Daniel Sommerhoff, Birgit J. Neuhaus, Ralf Schmidmaier, Stefan Ufer, and Tina Seidel

This chapter's simulation at a glance

Domain	Teacher education
Topic	Mathematical argumentation skills in the context of geometrical proofs
Learner's task	Taking on the role of pre-service interns and diagnosing the mathematical argumentation skills of four simulated seventh graders
Target group	Pre-service mathematic teachers
Diagnostic mode	Individual diagnosing
Sources of information	Interaction; observation of videos showing one-on-one student–teacher interactions
Special features	Simulated on-the-fly formative assessment situations

---

E. Codreanu (✉) · S. Huber
Department Educational Sciences, TUM School of Social Sciences and Technology, Technical University of Munich (TUM), Munich, Germany
e-mail: elias.codreanu@tum.de

S. Reinhold
Chair for Learning and Instruction, Center for International Student Assessment (ZIB), Technical University of Munich (TUM), Munich, Germany

D. Sommerhoff
Mathematics Education, IPN-Leibniz Institute for Science and Mathematics Education, Kiel, Germany

B. J. Neuhaus
Biology Education, Faculty for Biology, LMU Munich, Munich, Germany

R. Schmidmaier
Institute for Medical Education, University Hospital, LMU Munich, Munich, Germany

Department of Internal Medicine IV, University Hospital, LMU Munich, Munich, Germany

© The Author(s) 2022
F. Fischer, A. Opitz (eds.), *Learning to Diagnose with Simulations*,
https://doi.org/10.1007/978-3-030-89147-3_4

4.1 Diagnosing Based on Student Observation

Every day, teachers face a variety of diagnostic situations in which they gather information about their students' learning prerequisites, processes, and outcomes (Herppich et al., 2018; Praetorius et al., 2013; Ruiz-Primo & Furtak, 2007; Thiede et al., 2015). This information serves as a basis for different pedagogical decisions like lesson planning, adaptive teaching, or grading students (Schrader, 2013; Dünnebier et al., 2009; Südkamp et al., 2012; Vogt & Rogalla, 2009). In particular, diagnostic decisions are indispensable for the continuous, on-the-fly adaptation of one's teaching to students' individual needs and ongoing learning processes. Across educational systems, such diagnostic situations arise within the everyday student–teacher interactions that dominate classrooms (Klug et al., 2013; Furtak et al., 2016; Kingston & Nash, 2011; Birenbaum et al., 2006). Teachers require professional vision to glean significant information from these classroom situations and reason about them (Seidel & Stürmer, 2014). During such high-density interactions, they engage in describing, evaluating, and explaining in order to make meaningful decisions about pedagogical actions.

For pre-service teachers, these high-density interactions are often experienced as overwhelming, since they require the deliberate employment of diagnostic decision-making (Levin et al., 2009). Therefore, many pre-service teachers struggle to find their way around into the profession (Stokking et al., 2003). Nevertheless, diagnostic skills for diagnostic situations in the classroom are rarely taught in teacher education. Initially, university teacher education focuses on conveying basic principles and conceptual knowledge, often separated into different fields related to content knowledge, pedagogical content knowledge, and educational psychology. Given these structures, it is often unclear how these aspects of professional knowledge are related to specific diagnostic situations in classrooms (Alles et al., 2019). Therefore, new ways of supporting the acquisition of crucial skills like diagnostic skills are needed to prepare pre-service teachers to make reasonable diagnostic decisions before they enter their first classroom. Additionally, little is known about the processes involved in diagnostic decision-making and differences in these processes along the learning trajectory (Herppich et al., 2018). Insights into these processes may be promising to identify characteristics for targeted interventions along this learning trajectory.

S. Ufer
Chair of Mathematics Education, LMU Munich, Munich, Germany

T. Seidel
Friedl Schöller Endowed Chair for Educational Psychology, School of Education, Technical University of Munich (TUM), Munich, Germany

4.2 Simulation as a Model of Reality

An environment to investigate and promote pre-service teachers' diagnostic skills should encompass two aspects: First, following a practice-oriented approach, it should represent practice in an authentic way in order to motivate pre-service teachers to get involved in the actual task (Schubert et al., 2001). This, in turn, allows pre-service teachers to transfer their behavior from the simulated environment to real-world teaching situations. Second, reality must be decomposed and simplified in a way that enables pre-service teachers to focus on particular aspects of classroom situations (Grossman et al., 2009). Such decompositions of practice contain key features that make diagnostic decision-making more accessible to pre-service teachers than in real-world classroom situations.

Due to its strengths in both respects, video is becoming a frequently used medium in professional teacher education (Kang & van Es, 2018; Gaudin & Chaliès, 2015). Although videos can capture only one perspective on a classroom situation, and thus have a limited ability to convey the contextual background of the situation, videos can give authentic insights into different teaching and learning situations (Blomberg et al., 2013). Moreover, by taking a certain perspective, videos can direct observers' attention to significant features of the situation using so-called cues. Applying the idea of decomposing practice, in the specific sense of diagnosing students' skills based on observing them in the classroom, videos should capture everyday student-teacher interactions, including the most relevant cues for diagnosis but only a few less relevant cues that can distract teachers' attention in real-world classrooms. If the goal is to diagnose mathematical argumentation skills from a mathematics educational perspective, the most relevant cues include students' statements regarding their understanding of correct mathematical proof procedures, for example. General aspects like students' situational motivation can be considered less relevant for making such diagnoses. Reducing the number of less relevant cues increases teachers' capacity for deliberate action. The scripted video format also uniquely allows for further targeted manipulation of these segments (Piwowar et al., 2017).

Not just the makeup of scripted videos but also their embedding in a simulated environment influences learning grounded in practice. Decomposing the situation by dividing a scripted video into a number of scenes provides an opportunity to slow down the actual situation and thereby reduce the density of interactions. By decomposing situations, simulations provide researchers with insights into processes and allow for gathering data for further analyses of diagnostic skills. The results of such analyses may then help to develop future evidence-based interventions.

4.3 Mathematical Argumentation Skills

Mathematics is a relevant subject for studying diagnostic situations involving student–teacher interactions because the traditional initiation-response-feedback teaching discourse is the prevalent form of teacher–student dialogue (Lipowsky et al., 2009). In mathematics, as a proof-based science, working with mathematical argumentation as well as with proofs, as a special form of this argumentation fulfilling strict standards (Stylianides, 2007), is a crucial learning activity. Mastery of these skills is a central learning goal in many secondary school systems (Kultusministerkonferenz., 2012). However, empirical studies have repeatedly shown that students have substantial problems when attempting to construct a mathematical proof (Healy & Hoyles, 2000; Harel & Sowder, 1998). In particular, being able to successfully construct mathematical proofs depends on different individual prerequisites (Sommerhoff et al., 2015; Schoenfeld, 1992). These factors can be used in the diagnostic situation as indicators for diagnosing students' skills in working with argumentations and proofs. Ufer et al. (2008) and Sommerhoff et al. (2015) emphasize students' *mathematical content knowledge*, *methodological knowledge*, and *problem-solving strategies* as three important prerequisites. However, these three prerequisites can be divided into more specific components for use in the diagnostic process, as described in the following paragraph.

Mathematical content knowledge comprises three different sub-concepts (Weigand et al., 2014). First, knowledge of *concept properties* encompasses knowledge of features and terms, like features of the diagonals of parallelograms. The second sub-concept, known as *concept scope*, concerns knowledge of the entirety of representatives of a mathematical term. For example, this includes the knowledge that a square is a representative of the term parallelogram. Third, the *concept network* refers to knowledge about the relationship between a concept and other concepts. Likewise, methodological knowledge—that is, knowledge about the nature of proofs, their use within mathematics, and socio-mathematical norms regarding proofs—can be divided into at least three components (Heinze & Reiss, 2003): Knowledge of *proof scheme* encompasses knowledge about acceptable types of inferences in a proof. *Proof structure*, in contrast, refers to the overall logical structure of a proof, such as starting with assumptions and ending with an assertation. Finally, *chain of conclusion* refers to the logical arrangement of individual arguments within the proof. With respect to problem-solving strategies, this research project focuses on two different aspects. First, *heuristic strategies* help to solve a given problem task by reorganizing the task and changing how one looks at it. Second, *metacognitive strategies* allow an individual to control the problem-solving process through strategies such as monitoring and assessing their progress within the problem-solving process and drawing conclusions for action.

Prior research indicates that students typically differ widely regarding each of these eight aspects, resulting in a range of difficulties when attempting mathematical proofs (Reiss & Ufer, 2009). It is a difficult task for teachers to diagnose the reasons for students' difficulties and thus also what form of teacher support will help each individual student based solely on brief student–teacher interactions and possibly a brief look at students' notes.

4.4 Guiding Questions in Designing the Simulation

Both measuring and supporting teachers' diagnostic skills via simulations require high standards in terms of the simulations' authenticity and the content of the embedded videos. The development of the video-based simulation presented in this chapter was thus guided by the following questions (Codreanu et al., 2020):

1. To what extent can we authentically represent a diagnostic situation within student–teacher interaction around mathematical argumentation in a scripted video-based simulation?
2. To what extent can the decomposition of the diagnostic situation in the video-based simulation provide insights into the participants' diagnostic processes?

4.5 Conceptualization of the Scripted Videos

To create a simulated setting for diagnosing individual students' mathematical argumentation skills in a simulated classroom situation, we developed scripted videos with small-group student–teacher interactions, following Dieker et al. (2009)'s recommendations. First, we identified the essential features of the relevant situation (*selection of practice*). Second, we developed a contextual frame for all of the recordings as well as detailed scripts for each scene (*vignette script development*). Third, we created the video footage and edited it to create a representation of teaching practice (*video production*).

Selection of Practice We decided to focus on three individual student prerequisites that are important predictors of their performance when working with proofs (Ufer et al., 2008): (a) *mathematical content knowledge*, (b) *methodological knowledge*, and (c) *problem-solving strategies*. All three prerequisites have been shown to affect students' skills in working with geometrical proofs and can be portrayed in brief video clips. We considered the three sub-concepts of mathematical content knowledge, the three sub-concepts of methodological knowledge, and the two aspects of problem-solving strategies as a theoretical fundament when designing the student profiles.

Afterwards, we outlined four student profiles varying in their levels of the aforementioned prerequisites of students' skills in working with argumentations and proofs (eight aspects in total). Van Hiele's model of children's development of geometric thinking provided valuable additional guidance in this context (Usiskin, 1982). According to this model, a student on the first level can recognize and judge

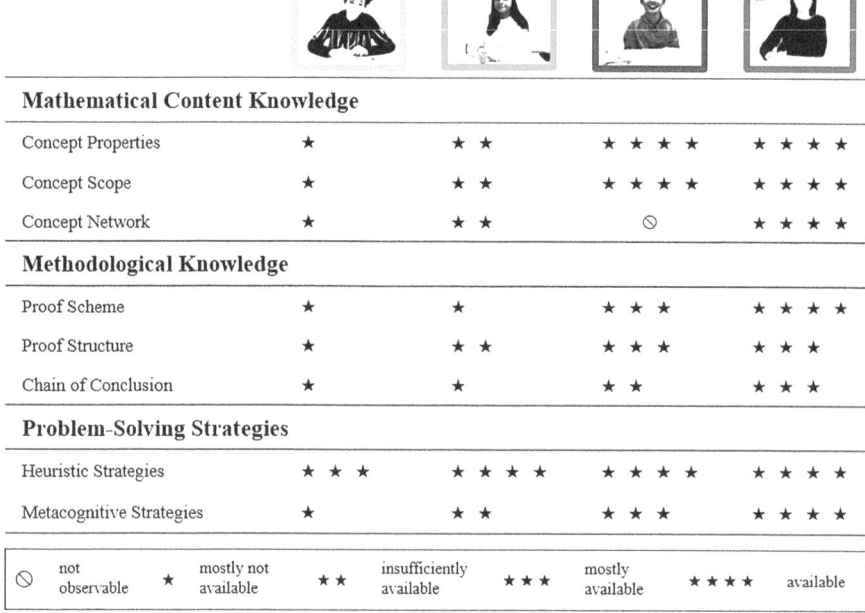

Fig. 4.1 Four student profiles and their specific predictive prerequisites for performance in working with proofs

figures by their appearance. A student on the second level can identify properties of figures, while a student on the third level can already follow simple deductions. Only at level four has a student acquired sufficient understanding to meaningfully construct proofs. We concentrated on these four levels and specified the student profiles based on their knowledge and abilities with respect to the eight predictive aspects. For example, Profiles A and B know little about what inferences are acceptable (*proof scheme*), whereas Profile C by and large and Profile D fully understand this point (see Fig. 4.1).

To ensure that the simulated students remained comparable, all simulated students worked on the same geometry proof task in the video clips: They had to prove that opposite sides of a parallelogram are of equal length, based on the information that pairs of sides of a parallelogram are parallel. Students who are just beginning to learn how to work with proofs do not pay a lot of attention to norms and standards of proofs on an abstract level. Thus, we did not expect all aspects, especially those for methodological knowledge, to become important in the proof construction process for these students. Likewise, it is possible that not all four simulated students need to use the conceptual network during the proof construction process. This is why we took care to select a task that can be completed in different ways to serve as a basis for the simulation.

Vignette Script Development for Staged Videos The time the simulated students spent working on the geometrical proof task was split into eight smaller video scenes, each with a length of approximately 1 min. Thus, all simulated students were depicted in the same number of scenes, which was sufficient to provide participants with the opportunity to observe each simulated student multiple times. The scripts for these scenes contained detailed dialogues between the teacher and simulated student, as well as copies of the simulated students' sketches and other notes in their exercise books. The teacher's input in the scenes was reduced to a minimum, focusing solely on eliciting the simulated students to talk about their thoughts. Thus, typical questions and requests by the teacher were "What do you mean by that?" or "Can you explain what you have done here?"

The answers and statements given by the simulated students were generated according to their profiles and under consideration of the eight identified aspects of predictive prerequisites. Cues could be found not only in the verbal teacher-student interaction but also in the students' sketches and notes. When creating the scenes, the cue attributions were continuously reviewed in an internal review process to ensure that the video scenes provided salient cues for the prerequisites. These cues were distributed as evenly as possible over the eight scenes in order to portray an authentic conversation. This resulted in a distribution in which at least one (and often more than one) salient cue for each aspect occurred no later than the fourth video scene.

Production of Staged Videos The video-recording was completed with one trained teacher and four eighth-grade student volunteers. The teacher and students were provided with the scripts prior to filming and were given time and guidance to familiarize themselves with their role, the script, and each other. While the scene between the teacher and one student was being filmed, the other students practiced their next scene with a member of the video production team. During shooting, the actors followed the scripts with as much fidelity as natural behavior allowed in that moment. The research team ensured that the main cues within the scripts were successfully captured on video. To capture both the verbal student–teacher interaction and the students' written notes, two different camera perspectives were used at the same time: One from the front showing the conversation, and one from above showing the student's exercise book. In the editing process, the scenes were cut to show the appropriate camera angle in each moment. After production was complete, the final video scenes were reviewed by two independent researchers with respect to the perceptibility of the cues contained in the initial scripts. In a subsequent consensus process based on the final video scenes, the four student profiles were classified into four ordinal categories with respect to each predictive prerequisite (see Fig. 4.1).

4.6 Design of the Simulation

The presented video-based simulation has an underlying structure consisting of four main parts (see Fig. 4.2). It starts by familiarizing participants with the situation depicted in the simulation, a pre-service intern observing student-teacher interactions during a student exercise concerning a geometric proof (*diagnostic situation*). Before participants start working with the tool, they are introduced to the task to be accomplished in this diagnostic situation: the simulated teacher asks them to assess the students' mathematical argumentation skills so that he can choose tasks for individual learning support in a subsequent class based on the participants' observations (*diagnostic task*). After that, participants can work independently in the simulated classroom situation to gather information about the students by watching the video scenes and taking notes (*diagnostic process*). These notes form the basis for the final diagnosis of each simulated student, which participants formulate in the last section of the tool to provide the simulated teacher a basis for his further lesson planning (*diagnostic outcome*).

Diagnostic Situation The situation chosen for this simulation is an everyday classroom situation in mathematics lessons (Lipowsky et al., 2009). Students are working independently on a task, in this case, a geometry proof, while the teacher walks from student to student to monitor and support their progress in short student-teacher interactions. At the beginning of the simulation, participants are familiarized with their role in this simulation: they are observing the teacher and students' interactions in their role as pre-service intern. In addition, they receive information about the overall topic, prior lessons, and learning context in order to acquaint them with the classroom situation as well as with the content discussed in the lesson. Taking on the role of an intern is familiar to participants (pre-service teachers), so they should be able to put themselves in this role without all too much effort. Thus, the scenario is likely to support immersion into the simulation (Slater & Wilbur, 1997). Furthermore, interns in real-life classrooms face similar challenges and opportunities to the ones contained in the diagnostic process later in the simulated situation. This parallelism between an intern's role in real-world situations and in the simulated diagnostic situation is expected to lead to higher authenticity of the learning environment (Schubert et al., 2001).

After the introduction to their role, participants receive information about the different steps a teacher considers when preparing a lesson. Information about the prior knowledge of the whole class and the topics covered in the class's previous lessons is provided. In addition, participants have an opportunity to familiarize themselves with the proof task for the upcoming lesson.

Diagnostic Task After familiarizing themselves with the diagnostic situation, the simulated teacher presents the diagnostic task to the participants. They are asked to diagnose four specific simulated students' level of understanding of working with geometric proofs in order to give the simulated teacher ideas for individual student support in a subsequent remedial lesson.

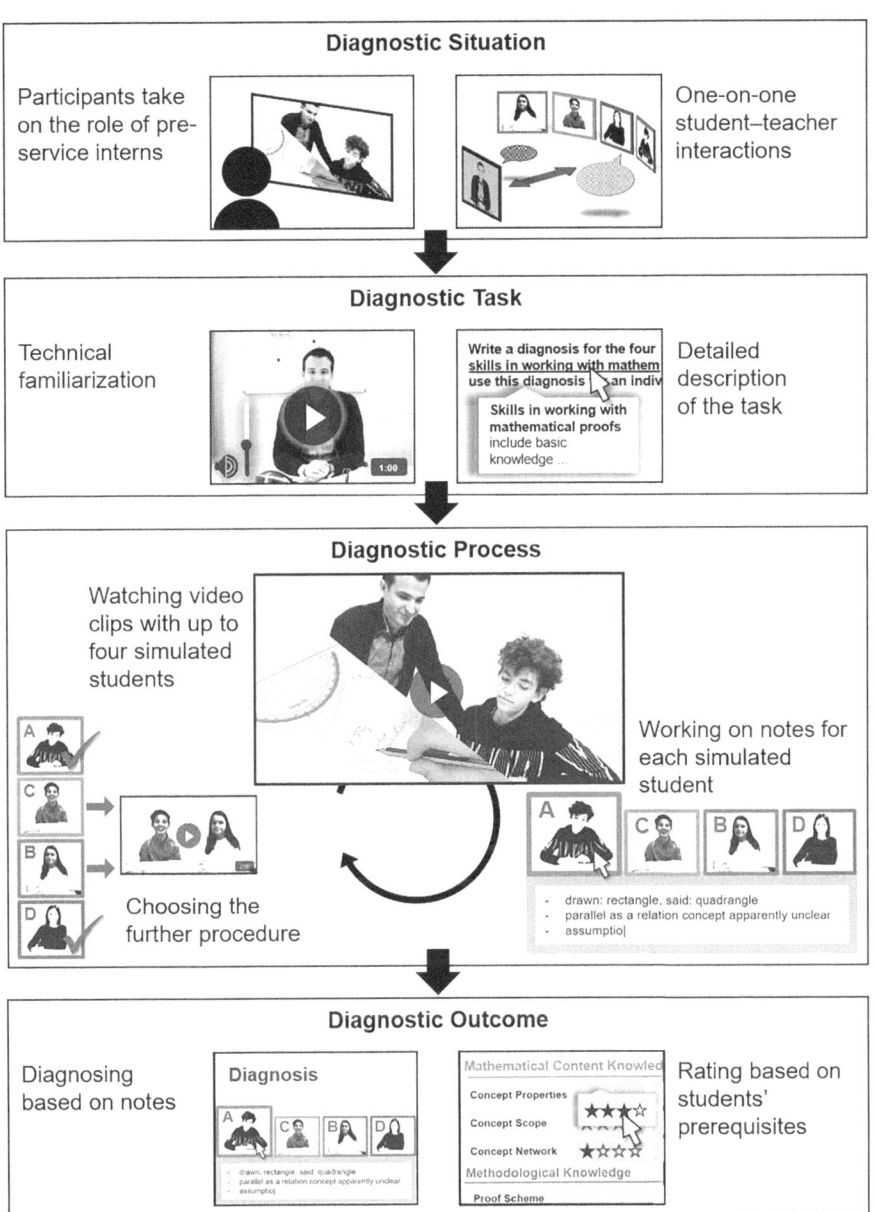

Fig. 4.2 Design of the video-based simulation. Note: Adapted from "Between authenticity and cognitive demand: Finding a balance in designing a video-based simulation in the context of mathematics teacher education" by Codreanu et al., 2020, *Teaching and Teacher Education*, 95, 103,146

We strive for two goals during the presentation of the diagnostic task: participants should come to understand both the specific task in detail and its embedding in the simulation. On the one hand, presenting the task during a short video clip familiarizes participants with the technical aspects of the simulation. For example, participants have the possibility to play and pause but not rewind the video in order to more closely simulate reality. This technical familiarization aims to minimize technical complications later in the diagnostic process. Additionally, participants get to know the teacher they will accompanying in the subsequent simulation. As a second major aim, the diagnostic task is described in detail, focusing on the following two aspects: (a) *who* is the diagnosis for and thus *how* should it look, and (b) what is the diagnosis' *purpose* and which *components* should it therefore entail? Considering that the participants most likely have little experience with diagnosing students' skills and abilities and the terminology used in this field, we provide a detailed description of the task to be completed in the subsequent diagnostic process. Regarding aspect (a), it is pointed out that a diagnosis should include descriptions, explanations, and decisions (Blömeke et al., 2015; Seidel & Stürmer, 2014). Regarding aspect (b), a description of the ability to work with geometrical proofs is provided, addressing the predictive prerequisites implemented in the video clips (see Fig. 4.1).

Diagnostic Process During the diagnostic process, the participants observe four simulated students, which simulates a reduced classroom setting. The process is divided into several cycles. Each cycle starts with watching one video clip containing student–teacher interaction scenes between one of the simulated students and the teacher. In the first cycle, participants observe all four simulated students in a row. Participants can take notes while observing the simulated students. Participants can enter their notes for each simulated student in the respective text box by clicking on the picture of each simulated student. This makes it possible to take individual notes for each simulated student. At the end of a cycle, participants must choose whether or not to continue the procedure. They can decide whether they want to observe more interactions with each student and thus run through another cycle of the diagnostic process for them, or conclude the diagnostic process for this particular simulated student. Thus, if a participant decides to continue observing two of the four simulated students, for example, the next cycle shows only these two students' further work on the proof task. Only the text boxes for the two remaining simulated students can be opened. After this second cycle has been completed, participants again decide whether to continue to observe each of the remaining simulated students in a third cycle. This continues until participants choose to conclude the observation process for all four simulated students or after a maximum of eight cycles.

In the first cycle, participants start with an empty text box for their note-taking. In subsequent cycles, notes from the previous cycles are already displayed in the text box, so that participants can further add to their previous notes. These notes serve as individual support to participants throughout the entire diagnostic process. However, the maximum number of scenes participants can watch is limited to 20. Thus, they must allocate the number of scenes they watch depicting each of the four simulated students. This also makes it possible to measure the efficiency of the participants' diagnostic process.

Diagnostic Outcome Finally, after participants complete the diagnostic process for all simulated students, they have to submit their diagnoses in two different ways. First, they are asked to formulate a diagnosis for each simulated student in an open-response text box. Their notes from the diagnostic process are shown above the text box. The participants can copy parts of the notes, summarize their points, or use the notes as an aid to remember the situations in the video clips. Like in the notes page, they can work on the four diagnoses in any order. Second, participants are asked to assess the simulated students' mathematical content knowledge, methodological knowledge, and problem-solving strategies. Participants have to rate the students' possession of each of the eight predictive prerequisites on a four-point Likert scale. These two tasks allow for participants' diagnostic outcomes to be assessed in two different ways, enabling a more differentiated consideration (see Fig. 4.1). Additionally, participants are asked to rank the student profiles according to their level of mathematical argumentation skills from weakest to strongest.

4.7 Discussion and Outlook

The video-based simulation developed in this project provides an innovative way to investigate and promote pre-service teachers' diagnostic skills regarding students' mathematical argumentation skills. The described development process is likely crucial for the effectiveness of video-based simulations targeting diagnostic skills in teacher education (see overarching research question 1 in Fischer et al., 2022). The purposeful conceptualization of the scripted videos and the simulation design suggest that the environment represents practice authentically and allows participants to immerse themselves in the situation. This supports the transfer of behavior to real-world situations. The specific facet of practice chosen for the scripted videos, namely the geometry task and student-teacher interactions surrounding it, resemble situations found in real-world mathematics classrooms. Moreover, the four meticulously designed student profiles capture important student prerequisites in terms of mathematical content knowledge, methodological knowledge, and problem-solving strategies (Ufer et al., 2008). Finally, the video clips were filmed with student volunteers, who enriched the script with their natural behavior. In the simulation itself, we separated the content-related and technical familiarization with the task from the part where the participants actually work on the simulation task. Hence, all information required to work undisturbed on the task and all additional instructions on the simulated situation are provided before the actual diagnostic process starts. This makes it possible to immerse oneself more deeply into the situation. In empirical analyses, expert teachers' and pre-service teachers' ratings of the authenticity and immersion of the scripted videos and the simulation as a whole are used to evaluate whether participants experience the simulated learning environment as a convincing representation of real-world classrooms (e.g. Codreanu et al., 2020). We involve expert teachers due to their wealth of experience in classroom situations, and novice teachers because they represent the target group for whom the simulation was developed. These and other variables are likely moderating and mediating variables for the successful completion of the simulation as well as embedding additional instructional support in the simulation (see overarching research question 3 in Fischer et al., 2022).

The specific conceptualization and design of the scripted videos and their embedding in the simulation both contribute to decomposing practice in a way that allows for the extraction of features regarding the participants' diagnostic process (see overarching research question 4 in Fischer et al., 2022). The scripted videos depict only four simulated students whose profiles differ only with regard to important prerequisites for successfully completing geometrical proofs. This makes it easier for participants to focus on and distinguish between students than in a classroom with twenty-plus students with more diverse compositions of those prerequisites. The deliberate absence of classroom management issues such as handling disturbances gives participants the opportunity to concentrate on more relevant rather than less relevant cues in their diagnostic processes. Adding time to the participants' observations by having them take notes slows down the ongoing classroom actions. While a real-world classroom does not include specific times to take notes on what teachers notice and interpret, the simulation does include these processes. Furthermore, the instructions to both describe and interpret one's observations in the notes helps teacher process in detail what they have observed. This reduces the complexity of the situation and allows participants to record important mental steps. Additionally, the notes give insight into participants' reasoning use and performance (Seidel & Stürmer, 2014). These data can help identify key features in the diagnostic process in order to develop targeted support within the simulation. Thus, analyzing pre-service teachers' diagnostic processes should reveal differences in where instructional support like scaffolding and prompts can be set (see overarching research question 2 in Fischer et al., 2022).

We expect to obtain further findings on the processes and variables that influence simulation performance by investigating participants' individual prerequisites, like their knowledge base or interest and self-concept. Based on these findings, the simulation will be expanded from a tool to assess diagnostic skills into a tool that is also able to foster those skills.

Acknowledgments The research presented in this chapter was funded by a grant from the Deutsche Forschungsgemeinschaft (DFG-FOR 2385) to Tina Seidel, Stefan Ufer, Birgit Neuhaus, and Ralf Schmidmaier (SE 1397/11-1).

References

Alles, M., Apel, J., Seidel, T., & Stürmer, K. (2019). How candidate teachers experience coherence in university education and teacher induction: The influence of perceived professional preparation at university and support during teacher induction. *Vocations and Learning, 12*, 87–112. https://doi.org/10.1007/s12186-018-9211-5

Birenbaum, M., Breuer, K., Cascallar, E., Dochy, F., Dori, Y., Ridgway, J., et al. (2006). A learning integrated assessment system. *Educational Research Review, 1*, 61–67. https://doi.org/10.1016/j.edurev.2006.01.001

Blomberg, G., Renkl, A., Sherin, M. G., Borko, H., & Seidel, T. (2013). Five research-based heuristics for using video in pre-service teacher education. *Journal of Educational Research Online, 5*(1), 90–114.

Blömeke, S., Gustafsson, J.-E., & Shavelson, R. J. (2015). Beyond dichotomies. *Zeitschrift für Psychologie, 223*, 3–13. https://doi.org/10.1027/2151-2604/a000194

Codreanu, E., Sommerhoff, D., Huber, S., Ufer, S., & Seidel, T. (2020). Between authenticity and cognitive demand: Finding a balance in designing a video-based simulation in the context of mathematics teacher education. *Teaching and Teacher Education, 95*, 103146. https://doi.org/10.1016/j.tate.2020.103146

Dieker, L. A., Lane, H. B., Allsopp, D. H., O'Brien, C., Butler, T. W., Kyger, M., et al. (2009). Evaluating video models of evidence-based instructional practices to enhance teacher learning. *Teacher Education and Special Education: The Journal of the Teacher Education Division of the Council for Exceptional Children, 32*, 180–196. https://doi.org/10.1177/0888406409334202

Dünnebier, K., Gräsel, C., & Krolak-Schwerdt, S. (2009). Urteilsverzerrungen in der schulischen Leistungsbeurteilung. *Zeitschrift für Pädagogische Psychologie, 23*, 187–195. https://doi.org/10.1024/1010-0652.23.34.187

Fischer, F., Chernikova, O., & Opitz, A. (2022). Learning to diagnose with simulations: Introduction. In F. Fischer & A. Opitz (Eds.), *Learning to diagnose with simulations – examples from teacher education and medical education*. Springer.

Furtak, E. M., Kiemer, K., Circi, R. K., Swanson, R., de León, V., Morrison, D., et al. (2016). Teachers' formative assessment abilities and their relationship to student learning: Findings from a four-year intervention study. *Instructional Science, 44*, 267–291. https://doi.org/10.1007/s11251-016-9371-3

Gaudin, C., & Chaliès, S. (2015). Video viewing in teacher education and professional development: A literature review. *Educational Research Review, 16*, 41–67. https://doi.org/10.1016/j.edurev.2015.06.001

Grossman, P., Compton, C., Igra, D., Ronfeldt, M., Shahan, E., & Williamson, P. W. (2009). Teaching practice: A cross-professional perspective. *Teachers College Record, 111*(9), 2055–2100.

Harel, G., & Sowder, L. (1998). Students' proof schemes: Results from exploratory studies. *CBMS Issues in Mathematics Education, 7*, 234–283.

Healy, L., & Hoyles, C. (2000). A study of proof conceptions in algebra. *Journal for Research in Mathematics Education, 31*(4), 396–428.

Heinze, A., & Reiss, K. (2003). Reasoning and proof: methodological knowledge as a component of proof competence. www.lettredelapreuve.itlCERME3PapersiHeinze-paperl.pdf.

Herppich, S., Praetorius, A.-K., Förster, N., Glogger-Frey, I., Karst, K., Leutner, D., et al. (2018). Teachers' assessment competence: Integrating knowledge-, process-, and product-oriented approaches into a competence-oriented conceptual model. *Teaching and Teacher Education, 76*, 181–193. https://doi.org/10.1016/j.tate.2017.12.001

Kang, H., & van Es, E. A. (2018). Articulating design principles for productive use of video in preservice education. *Journal of Teacher Education, 5*, 1–14. https://doi.org/10.1177/0022487118778549

Kingston, N., & Nash, B. (2011). Formative assessment: A meta-analysis and a call for research. *Educational Measurement: Issues and Practice, 30*, 28–37. https://doi.org/10.1111/j.1745-3992.2011.00220.x

Klug, J., Bruder, S., Kelava, A., Spiel, C., & Schmitz, B. (2013). Diagnostic competence of teachers: A process model that accounts for diagnosing learning behavior tested by means of a case scenario. *Teaching and Teacher Education, 30*, 38–46. https://doi.org/10.1016/j.tate.2012.10.004

Kultusministerkonferenz. (2012). *Bildungsstandards im Fach Mathematik für die allgemeine Hochschulreife*. KMK.

Levin, D. M., Hammer, D., & Coffey, J. E. (2009). Novice teachers' attention to student thinking. *Journal of Teacher Education, 60*, 142–154. https://doi.org/10.1177/0022487108330245

Lipowsky, F., Rakoczy, K., Pauli, C., Drollinger-Vetter, B., Klieme, E., & Reusser, K. (2009). Quality of geometry instruction and its short-term impact on students' understanding of the Pythagorean theorem. *Learning and Instruction, 19*, 527–537. https://doi.org/10.1016/j.learninstruc.2008.11.001

Piwowar, V., Barth, V. L., Ophardt, D., & Thiel, F. (2017). Evidence-based scripted videos on handling student misbehavior: The development and evaluation of video cases for teacher education. *Professional Development in Education, 44*, 369–384. https://doi.org/10.1080/19415257.2017.1316299

Praetorius, A.-K., Berner, V.-D., Zeinz, H., Scheunpflug, A., & Dresel, M. (2013). Judgment confidence and judgment accuracy of teachers in judging self-concepts of students. *The Journal of Educational Research, 106*, 64–76. https://doi.org/10.1080/00220671.2012.667010

Reiss, K., & Ufer, S. (2009). Was macht mathematisches Arbeiten aus? Empirische Ergebnisse zum Argumentieren, Begründen und Beweisen. *Jahresbericht der Deutschen Mathematiker-Vereinigung, 111*(4), 1–23.

Ruiz-Primo, M. A., & Furtak, E. M. (2007). Exploring teachers' informal formative assessment practices and students' understanding in the context of scientific inquiry. *Journal of Research in Science Teaching, 44*, 57–84. https://doi.org/10.1002/tea.20163

Schoenfeld, A. H. (1992). Learning to think mathematically: Problem solving, metacogntion, and sense making in mathematics. In D. Grouws (Ed.), *Handbook of research on mathematics teaching and learning* (pp. 334–370). Simon & Schuster.

Schrader, F.-W. (2013). Diagnostische Kompetenz von Lehrpersonen. *Beiträge zur Lehrerbildung, 31*(2), 154–165.

Schubert, T., Friedmann, F., & Regenbrecht, H. (2001). The experience of presence: Factor analytic insights. *Presence, 10*(3), 266–281.

Seidel, T., & Stürmer, K. (2014). Modeling and measuring the structure of professional vision in preservice teachers. *American Educational Research Journal, 51*, 739–771. https://doi.org/10.3102/0002831214531321

Slater, M., & Wilbur, S. (1997). A framework for immersive virtual environments (FIVE): Speculations on the role of presence in virtual environments. *Presence: Teleoperators and Virtual Environments, 6*(6), 603–616.

Sommerhoff, D., Ufer, S., & Kollar, I. (2015). Research on mathematical argumentation: A descriptive review of PME proceedings. In K. Beswick, T. Muir, & J. Wells (Eds.), *Proceedings of 39th Psychology of Mathematics Education conference* (pp. 193–200). PME.

Stokking, K., Leenders, F., de Jong, J., & van Tartwijk, J. (2003). From student to teacher: Reducing practice shock and early dropout in the teaching profession. *European Journal of Teacher Education, 26*, 329–350. https://doi.org/10.1080/0261976032000128175

Stylianides, A. J. (2007). Proof and proving in school mathematics. *Journal for Research in Mathematics Education, 38*(3), 289–321.

Südkamp, A., Kaiser, J., & Möller, J. (2012). Accuracy of teachers' judgments of students' academic achievement: A meta-analysis. *Journal of Educational Psychology, 104*, 743–762. https://doi.org/10.1037/a0027627

Südkamp, A., & Praetorius, A.-K. (2017). *Diagnostische Kompetenz von Lehrkräften: Theoretische und methodische Weiterentwicklungen (Pädagogische Psychologie und Entwicklungspsychologie)* (Vol. 94). Waxmann.

Thiede, K. W., Brendefur, J. L., Osguthorpe, R. D., Carney, M. B., Bremner, A., Strother, S., et al. (2015). Can teachers accurately predict student performance? *Teaching and Teacher Education, 49*, 36–44. https://doi.org/10.1016/j.tate.2015.01.012

Ufer, S., Heinze, A., & Reiss, K. (2008). Individual predictors of geometrical proof competence. *PME 32 and PME-NA XXX, 1*(4), 361–368.

Usiskin, Z. (1982). Van Hiele levels and achievement in secondary school geometry: CDASSG Project.

Vogt, F., & Rogalla, M. (2009). Developing adaptive teaching competency through coaching. *Teaching and Teacher Education, 25*, 1051–1060. https://doi.org/10.1016/j.tate.2009.04.002

Weigand, H.-G., Filler, A., Hölzl, R., Kuntze, S., Ludwig, M., Roth, J., et al. (2014). Didaktik der Geometrie für die Sekundarstufe I. In *Mathematik Primarstufe und Sekundarstufe I + II* (2nd ed.). Springer Spektrum.

Open Access This chapter is licensed under the terms of the Creative Commons Attribution 4.0 International License (http://creativecommons.org/licenses/by/4.0/), which permits use, sharing, adaptation, distribution and reproduction in any medium or format, as long as you give appropriate credit to the original author(s) and the source, provide a link to the Creative Commons license and indicate if changes were made.

The images or other third party material in this chapter are included in the chapter's Creative Commons license, unless indicated otherwise in a credit line to the material. If material is not included in the chapter's Creative Commons license and your intended use is not permitted by statutory regulation or exceeds the permitted use, you will need to obtain permission directly from the copyright holder.

Chapter 5
Diagnosing 6th Graders' Understanding of Decimal Fractions: Fostering Mathematics Pre-Service Teachers' Diagnostic Competences with Simulated One-on-One Interviews

Bernhard Marczynski, Larissa J. Kaltefleiter, Matthias Siebeck, Christof Wecker, Kathleen Stürmer, and Stefan Ufer

This chapter's simulation at a glance

Domain	Teacher education
Topic	Diagnosing student understanding and misconceptions of decimal fractions
Learner's task	Taking on the role of a teacher, student, or observer during a (simulated) diagnostic task-based interview on decimal fractions
Target group	Mathematics teacher education students with some prior pedagogical content knowledge of decimal fractions
Diagnostic mode	Individual diagnosis by teachers
Sources of information	Teacher–student interaction based on diagnostic tasks
Special features	Based on current research on students' understanding of decimal fractions; trained actors or peer students as standardized students in a role-play simulation

---

B. Marczynski · L. J. Kaltefleiter · S. Ufer (✉)
Chair of Mathematics Education, LMU Munich, Munich, Germany
e-mail: ufer@math.lmu.de

M. Siebeck
Institute of Medical Education, University Hospital, LMU Munich, Munich, Germany

Department of General, Visceral und Transplantation Surgery, University Hospital, LMU Munich, Munich, Germany

© The Author(s) 2022
F. Fischer, A. Opitz (eds.), *Learning to Diagnose with Simulations*,
https://doi.org/10.1007/978-3-030-89147-3_5

5.1 Introduction

5.1.1 Diagnosing Mathematical Understanding in Direct Teacher–Student Interaction

Results from educational research emphasize the importance of teachers' diagnostic competences for adaptive teaching and thus for improved student learning (e.g., Behrmann & Souvignier, 2013). Consequently, teacher training standards (e.g., KMK, 2004) highlight diagnostic competences as a central goal of teacher education at university. This, in turn, results in a need for evidence-based training methods.

Diagnosing is understood here as the goal-directed accumulation and integration of information to reduce uncertainty when making educational decisions (cf. Heitzmann et al., 2019) such as adaptive teaching, lesson planning, or student assessment (Schrader, 2013). While previous research has focused on judgment accuracy (i.e., the match between teachers' expectation concerning a student's performance on a test and that student's actual performance on that test; Spinath, 2005), recent work suggests the need to include more qualitative evaluations of the learner's understanding, misconceptions, and strategies (e.g., Herppich et al., 2017) and to also study the diagnostic process that leads to teachers' judgments.

We conceptualize diagnostic competences as the collection of teachers' individual resources that enable them to attend to and interpret students' mathematical thinking in a variety of situations (Jacobs et al., 2010; Nickerson et al., 2017; Weinert, 2001). While diagnostic situations in teachers' practice may vary substantially (Karst et al., 2017), most arise within student-teacher interactions in the classroom (Klug et al., 2013), have the formative assessment of student learning as their goal, and are closely intertwined with the teacher's pedagogical actions (Kaiser et al., 2017).

Based on the above definition, the accuracy and effectiveness of teachers' diagnoses in a range of situations—in terms of reducing the uncertainty of the pedagogical decision at hand—serves as the primary indicator for observing diagnostic competences. However, indicators from the diagnostic process itself might also provide insights into a teacher's diagnostic competences. Firstly, it might be considered to what extent a teacher's interaction with a student is indeed suited to generate interpretable evidence about students' mathematical thinking, for example, by posing diagnostically rich ("probing") questions (van den Kieboom et al., 2014). On the other hand, research on teachers' noticing suggests that it would be worthwhile to examine the depth with which teachers process their observations during

---

C. Wecker
Institute of Education, University of Hildesheim, Hildesheim, Germany

K. Stürmer
Hector Research Institute of Education Sciences and Psychology, University of Tübingen, Tübingen, Germany

diagnosing. Seidel and Stürmer (2014), for example, propose to differentiate between the mere *description* of relevant aspects of a situation "without making any further judgements" (p. 745); *explanations,* in which teachers link their observations to concepts and theories from their professional knowledge; and *predictions*, in which teachers draw conclusions about the consequences of the "observed events in terms of student learning" (p. 746).

Despite some first results from interventions fostering in-service teachers' judgment accuracy (e.g., Thiede et al., 2018), research that focuses on pre-service teachers, takes a broader view of diagnostic competences, and examines the role of characteristics of the diagnostic process for the final diagnosis as well as for development of diagnostic competences is still sparse.

5.1.2 *Role-Play-Based Simulations to Foster Diagnostic Competences*

University-based teacher education has traditionally put an emphasis on conveying professional knowledge, which is assumed to underlie competences such as diagnostic competences. Professional knowledge is often differentiated into content knowledge, pedagogical content knowledge, and pedagogical knowledge (e.g., Kleickmann et al., 2012). Based on the assumption that "integration is simple and builds up automatically" (Harr et al., 2014, p. 1), these knowledge domains are often taught separately, thus leaving "the challenge of integration to the individual teacher" (Harr et al., 2014, p. 1). Additionally, content from these knowledge domains is first encoded as declarative knowledge, but practice is an essential prerequisite for the transformation of this declarative content into procedural knowledge and skills (Anderson, 1982, 1987). However, many teacher education programs seem to lack this linkage between knowledge acquisition and practice (Beck & Kosnik, 2002; Fraser, 2007). As a result, weak connections between the knowledge domains are frequent, and pre-service teachers are likely to struggle to use this knowledge in practice (Alles et al., 2018).

In the same vein, Shavelson (2012) proposes using "holistic, real-world problems" (p. 58) to assess competences such as diagnosing. He mentions both task authenticity (e.g., Seidel et al., 2010) and the feeling of immersion into the task situation ("presence," cf. Schubert et al., 2001, pp. 266ff.; Frank, 2015) as characteristics of valid learning and assessment tasks. However, situations involving diagnosis in everyday teacher practice are often characterized by a complex interaction between managing student-teacher interactions, making diagnoses, making pedagogical decisions, and enacting pedagogical interventions. This complexity may overstrain unexperienced learners and impede their learning. If such situations are included in early phases of teacher education, a central problem is to find a balance between tasks' authenticity and their complexity (Seidel et al., 2015).

Therefore, Grossman et al. (2009b) propose a "*decomposition of practice*" into its basic components in order to reduce complexity and so-called *approximations of practice*, which enable pre-service teachers "to engage in practices that are more or less proximal to the practices" (p. 2056) of their future profession. Based on the above, Seidel et al. (2015) provide a differential clarification of the relation between these two goals:

> "Novices are faced with a myriad factors to be taken into account in the initial experiences of teaching. Thus, the acquisition of professional practice is not characterized by simply increasing the quantity of classroom teaching practice – the most complex form of teaching practice – but by building up a series of approximations to a practice that increases in complexity and that allows for systematically linking elements of professional knowledge to corresponding elements in professional practice." (p. 86)

Similar to this idea, using diagnostic interviews to separate diagnostic demands from pedagogical decision-making and practice in *initial* teacher education has been proposed repeatedly in the past (Grossman et al., 2009a; Schack et al., 2013) and may be one form of *decomposition*. Furthermore, simulations of such interviews, e.g., in the form of role-plays, may provide an effective way to control complexity in this kind of learning situation. However, knowledge of learning processes in such simulations and factors influencing their effectiveness in initial teacher education is still scarce, and numerous research gaps exist regarding how these competences can be supported through instruction. Consequently, research on feasible and efficient learning environments to help mathematics pre-service teachers acquire those competences seems to be justified.

Medical education has recently studied role-play-based simulations as learning environments (e.g., Lane et al., 2008; Stegmann et al., 2012), and has also addressed their potential feasibility and benefits for teacher education (Gartmeier et al., 2015). Within the context of those studies, role-play-based simulations have proven an effective means of fostering communicative competences, especially during early phases of their acquisition (Berkhof et al., 2011; Lane & Rollnick, 2007). Further studies indicate that learning by observation and active role-taking (e.g., Stegmann et al., 2012) may foster the acquisition of competences within such simulations.

5.2 A Role-Play-Based Simulation of Diagnostic One-on-One Interviews

This chapter presents the conceptualization and development of a role-play-based simulation of one-on-one diagnostic interviews in DiMaL, a project that aims to study pre-service teachers' learning processes in such simulations and their effects in university-based pre-service teacher education.

5.2.1 Selection of the Diagnostic Situation

In line with prior approaches to fostering pre-service teachers' diagnostic competences (McDonough et al., 2002), and to ensure that the simulated interviews will successfully target central aspects of diagnostic competence as part of pre-service teachers' training, it was necessary for the simulations to represent real-life job demands (Shavelson, 2012). Therefore, we focused on decimal fractions as the interview content. Research on students' errors and misconceptions regarding decimals has a long tradition in mathematics education (Brueckner, 1928; Heckmann, 2006; Steinle, 2004) and is addressed in university-based teacher education in many countries (e.g., Lortie-Forgues et al., 2015; Ministry of Education, 2008; Padberg & Wartha, 2017). We placed focus on three areas of knowledge of decimal fractions that have been reported as particularly difficult in the past:

1. Principles of number representation in the decimal place value system, including the application to comparing decimals.
2. Flexible and adaptive use of calculation strategies for all four basic arithmetic operations.
3. The meaning of basic arithmetic operations One-on-one diagnostic interviews diagnostic situation in real-world situations (e.g., partitive and quotative situations for division by rational numbers).

5.2.2 Use Scenarios for the Simulation

Simulations, as approximations of practice, may serve as learning opportunities within teacher education (Grossman et al., 2009a), but can also deliver formative and summative information about pre-service teachers' diagnostic competences (Shavelson, 2012). When developing the simulation, we anticipated two different use scenarios:

In a *learning scenario*, the simulation serves as an approximation of practice to support meaningful learning in university-based teacher education. In this scenario, participants engaging in the simulation take on one of three roles: One participant acts in the teacher role, while a second participant takes on the role of the simulated student (grade 6). A third participant may take on the role of an observer (cf. Stegmann et al., 2012) who watches and reflects on the diagnostic interview enacted by the participants in the other two roles.

In an *assessment scenario*, the goal of the simulation is to derive information about pre-service teachers' diagnostic competences from the diagnostic process as well as the final diagnosis proposed. In this scenario, all participants take on the teacher role. For standardization purposes, the student role can be played by teacher education students who are specially trained to act as standardized sixth graders during the simulation. Apart from the standardization of the student role, the simulation follows the same procedure in both use scenarios.

5.2.3 Overview of the Simulation

We decided to construct an interactive role-play-based live simulation to approximate the diagnostic situation without too many restrictions on teachers' questions and simulated sixth graders' responses. Based on experiences with live simulations in medical education and teacher education (e.g., Gartmeier et al., 2015; Stegmann et al., 2012), the simulation was developed in close collaboration with a partner project from medical education (cf. Chap. 9).

A preparation phase for the simulation (15 min., cf. Fig. 5.1) acquaints participants with the technical aspects of the simulation and with the relevant content for their role. Participants in the teacher role study a set of diagnostic tasks that they can use during the interview, those in the student role study a description of the case profile they will enact later, and those in the observer role study an observation script. All participants can make notes for each task. A "fiction contract" informs participants about the natural restrictions of a simulation setting and asks them to engage in the simulation as they would in a comparable real interview as much as possible.

In the subsequent interview phase (30 min., cf. Fig. 5.1), participants in the teacher and student roles engage in the role-play-based simulation of the diagnostic interview, starting with a short introductory dialogue. The participant in the teacher role selects tasks, presents them to the simulated student, observes the answer, and has the opportunity to ask further probing questions. The participant in the teacher role is instructed to start the interview by selecting at least one sub-task from each of three initial *screening tasks*. Before they proceed to subsequent tasks, they are asked to provide an intermediate diagnosis. The participant in the student role works on the tasks as described in their case profile, while the participant in the observer role watches and analyzes the simulated interview using the observation script. Participants in the teacher and observer roles can take notes.

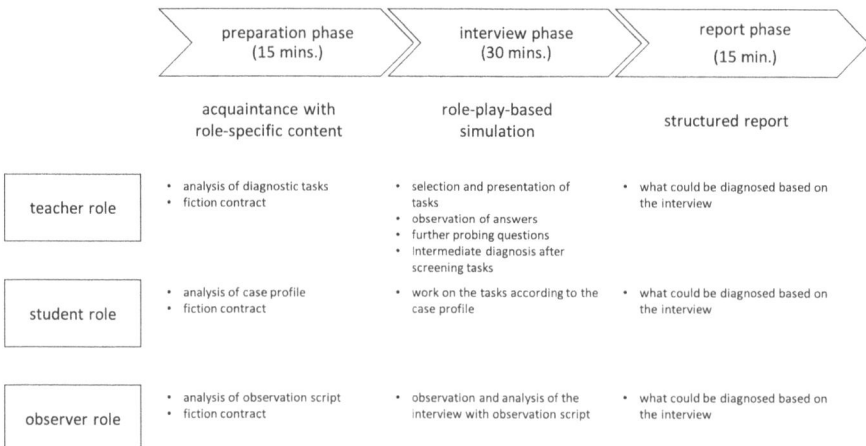

Fig. 5.1 Overview of content and tasks for each role in the simulation phase

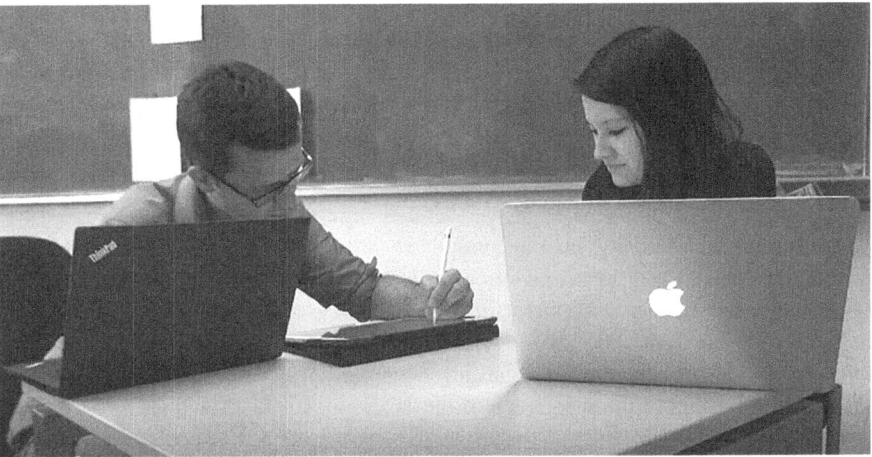

Fig. 5.2 Setup of the simulation environment from the observer's perspective, showing the student (left) and the teacher (right)

During the final report phase (15 min., cf. Fig. 5.1), participants in all three roles are asked to individually compose a structured report diagnosing the simulated student's knowledge and misconceptions based on the preceding interview. Participants in the student and observer roles are asked to take the perspective of the interviewer here, and to interpret the interview from this perspective.

Participants are guided through the simulation using a web-based simulation environment. During the interview phase, the participant in the interviewer role selects tasks from his or her computer screen (on the right-hand side of Fig. 5.2), while the participant in the student role can see the case profile on his or her own computer screen (on the left side of Fig. 5.2). The participant in the observer role can see the observation script. Moreover, there are text fields for the interviewer and the observer to take notes during the interview. Whenever the interviewer selects a task, the student's solution based on his or her case profile is displayed on the student's screen. The tasks are also presented on a tablet PC in the center of the setup, and the student solves the tasks by writing on the tablet PC with a digital pen (see the middle of Fig. 5.2). The tablet PC also records what is on its own screen and the verbal discourse during the simulation.

5.2.4 Development of Simulation Materials

Diagnostic Tasks Based on prior research on students' understanding of decimal fractions (e.g., Steinle, 2004), we designed a set of 16 diagnostic tasks for the simulation. Some tasks are diagnostically sensitive to typical errors and misconceptions, while other tasks can be solved without deeper understanding of decimals. The first three tasks are *screening tasks* that address one of the three main areas of knowledge regarding decimals. Each of these *screening tasks* contains some sub-tasks that are diagnostically sensitive and some sub-tasks that are not. The subsequent tasks may provide additional information for each of the main areas of decimal knowledge and can be selected freely by the interviewer after completion of the screening tasks.

Case Profiles In order to address knowledge and misconceptions in each of the three areas of decimal knowledge, we defined four student case profiles based on prior research on students' misconceptions regarding decimal fractions. Each case profile includes strong misconceptions about decimal fractions in one area of knowledge, partial misconceptions in a second area, and quite robust knowledge in the remaining area. The profiles contain detailed descriptions of the students' knowledge and misconceptions regarding decimals. A student solution and student justification for this solution for each of the 16 diagnostic tasks and each of the four case profiles were constructed that reflected each student's specific case profile. These solutions and justifications are displayed to the participant in the student role during the interview whenever a task is selected by the interviewer.

Structured Report Format Three different prompts were designed to obtain participants' final diagnoses. As a first rough diagnosis, participants are asked to enter a main and two alternative short descriptions of the student's main problems and provide information about their certainty in their diagnosis. The second prompt asks for a more extensive report to be given to the "teacher" of the simulated student, highlighting the students' understanding, misconceptions, and first ideas for specific instructional support for this student. Based on the concept of professional vision (e.g., Seidel & Stürmer, 2014; van Es & Sherin, 2002), participants are instructed to describe what they have observed during the interview, to explain their observations using knowledge from their university courses, and to predict possible consequences. The third prompt requires participants to judge to what extent the simulated student has mastered each of the three areas of knowledge on decimals in a closed answer format.

5.2.5 *Training Actors to Play Standardized Students*

When using the simulation to assess participants' diagnostic competences, having the simulated students act in a standardized way based on the case profiles becomes crucial. To achieve this, the pre-service teachers working as standardized students received a 10-hour acting training in three sessions. The training concept was based on prior research on micro-teaching events (Seidel et al., 2015) and role-play simulations in medicine (Stegmann et al., 2012). After a brief introduction to misconceptions on decimals and diagnosing mathematics skills, the actors were introduced to the interview setting, the technical environment and the diagnostic tasks, and the case profiles. Before the second session, they studied the case profiles in detail. The second session contained an active training with three diagnostic interviews, feedback by the project staff, and discussion of challenges and uncertainties in playing the simulated students. The third session comprised two test simulations in which a member of the project staff played the interviewer and provided feedback to the actors based on video recordings of the simulation. The training sought to maximize the simulation's authenticity and ensure an accurate depiction of the case profiles.

5.2.6 *Measures Derived from the Simulation*

Diagnostic Process The simulation offers three ways to gather data on the interviewer's diagnostic activities (Fischer et al., 2014) within the simulation. (1) The diagnostic sensitivity of the sub-tasks selected by the interviewer from the *screening tasks* serves as a measure of how well participants in the teacher role *generate diagnostic evidence*. (2) Analyzing to what extent participants in the teacher and observer roles describe, explain or predict based on their observations relates to the diagnostic activities of *evaluating evidence* and *drawing conclusions*. It also enables an analysis of how deeply participants process the diagnostic evidence (Seidel & Stürmer, 2014; van Es & Sherin, 2002). (3) Participants in the teacher role may pose verbal questions to their simulated students to elicit information about their mathematical thinking. The extent to which these questions allow participants to infer students' knowledge of decimals relates to the interviewers' *evidence generation*, but also involves the *creation of artifacts* (tasks and questions).

Diagnostic Product The diagnoses included in the final report provide information about the accuracy of the diagnosis, i.e., its match to the actual student profile. Moreover, the certainty ratings after the screening tasks and during the report phase allow this accuracy is accuracy to be related to the reduction of uncertainty during the diagnostic process. Finally, the descriptions, explanations, and predictions in the participants' written reports show how deeply the participants process diagnostic information when *communicating and scrutinizing* their conclusions.

5.3 Ensuring a Suitable Approximation of Practice

In order to ensure that the simulation can serve as an appropriate approximation of practice for learning and assessment at university, three aspects are currently under study. The associated studies focus on the assessment use case for the simulation.

Usability of the Simulation A pilot study with $N = 6$ mathematics pre-service teachers as participants was conducted. In the experimental session, the participants completed the whole simulation as described above twice; the case profiles were randomly assigned. Based on this pilot, several technical changes were made to the simulation platform to increase the usability of the system. For example, it turned out that some interviewers attempted to inform the simulated students about the correct solutions to the tasks (cf. van den Kieboom et al., 2014 for similar results). On the one hand, this may reflect high immersion into the simulation's diagnostic task and an experience of authenticity, which have been put forward as important characteristics of valid learning and assessment tasks (cf. Shavelson, 2012). On the other hand, focusing on instruction instead of diagnosis might decrease the learning opportunities for diagnostic competencies. For this reason, we included an additional button titled "explanation alert" on the student's computer screen in the interview system. If the interviewer starts to provide an explanation, the participant in the student role can select this button; after a certain amount of time, a warning message appears on the interviewer's screen instructing them to remember that their goal is to diagnose students' understanding.

Content of the Simulation Materials We are conducting a video-based survey among experts in mathematics education and educational sciences to obtain evaluations of the diagnostic tasks and case profiles included in the simulation. This includes the comprehensibility of the instructions given to the interviewer role, the authenticity of the case profiles, and the standardized implementation of these case profiles by the trained pre-service teachers.

Participants' Perception of the Simulated Situation As Shavelson (2012) highlights the importance of task authenticity and the experience of immersion into the task situation resulting from the simulation environment as characteristics of valid assessment and learning tasks, we will investigate these factors in a first validation study with mathematics pre-service teachers and practicing mathematics teachers. Using adaptations of established scales (Frank, 2015; Seidel et al., 2010), we will study participants' perception of authenticity and presence during the interview.

5.4 Conclusions and Outlook

In this chapter, we presented the conceptualization and development of a simulation that combines and extends three lines of research: Firstly, the simulation goes beyond the traditional conceptualization of teachers' diagnostic competences as judgment accuracy (Spinath, 2005) by including process features (Herppich et al., 2017). Based on data from the simulated diagnostic interviews, it is possible to describe both diagnostic processes during the interview and products of the diagnostic process. Secondly, the interviews are implemented as role-play-based simulations and represent approximations of practice focusing on a separable facet of teachers' professional work. Such a decomposition has been proposed for early phases of teacher education in particular (Grossman et al., 2009a). Thirdly, and in order to address the first two points, we make use of results from a long tradition of research on students' misconceptions of decimal fractions (e.g., Brueckner, 1928; Steinle, 2004). Prior research has also shown that mastering professional demands in one-on-one interviews such as those in our simulation poses a challenge to beginning mathematics teachers. Such demands include, for example, selecting diagnostically sensitive tasks or asking rich "probing" questions (van den Kieboom et al., 2014).

One main feature of the simulation is that it is developed for two different use scenarios: assessment and learning. The use of authentic and realistic tasks has been put forward in the literature as a criterion for valid assessment in higher education (Shavelson, 2012), making it desirable to study their added value beyond traditional paper-and-pencil-based assessments in teacher education. Moreover, such simulations have been proposed as a means to transform teacher education to focus more on teachers' professional tasks as a means of learning and applying professional knowledge (Grossman et al., 2009a).

Studying the suitability and effects of simulations for these two scenarios is the main goal of the DiMaL project. This will be addressed in further studies, including an expert survey to evaluate the diagnostic tasks, instructions, case profiles, and their implementation in terms of comprehensibility, authenticity, and standardization. Further studies will also focus on participants' perception of the simulated situation in terms of authenticity and immersion into the diagnostic task (Shavelson, 2012). Moreover, relations between pre-service teachers' professional knowledge, characteristics of their diagnostic process, and the accuracy and effectiveness of their diagnoses will be studied.

Nevertheless, the implementation of such simulations in pre-service teacher education still leaves a set of open questions. Despite the added value of such simulations over more traditional forms of instruction, open questions remain regarding the effects of the specific role taken within the simulation (teacher, student, or observer) on students' learning (cf. Stegmann et al., 2012 for medical diagnosis). Moreover, research from other fields has highlighted the need for reflection in order to learn from such simulations (e.g., Mamede et al., 2012, 2014). Future studies will address the four questions introduced by Fischer, Chernikova & Opitz (2022) and Opitz et al. (2022). To optimize learning (overarching research question 2), we will investigate a video-based implementation of the simulation, which will provide more guidance and structure than the role-play simulation, as well as additional support in the form of reflection prompts and knowledge activation prompts during the simulation. Moderation effects by prior knowledge on the effects of these scaffolds will be investigated (overarching research question 3). Together with an in-depth investigation of learning process measures (overarching research question 1), the results will be used to implement adaptive support for the two scaffolds (overarching research question 4).

Acknowledgments The research presented in this chapter was funded by a grant from the Deutsche Forschungsgemeinschaft (DFG-FOR 2385) to Stefan Ufer, Kathleen Stürmer, Christof Wecker, and Matthias Siebeck (UF59/5-1).

References

Alles, M., Apel, J., Seidel, T., & Stürmer, K. (2018). How candidate teachers experience coherence in university education and teacher induction: The influence of perceived professional preparation at university and support during teacher induction. *Vocations and Learning, 12*(1), 87–112. https://doi.org/10.1007/s12186-018-9211-5

Anderson, J. R. (1982). Acquisition of cognitive skill. *Psychological Review, 89*(4), 369–406. https://doi.org/10.1037/0033-295X.89.4.369

Anderson, J. R. (1987). Skill acquisition: Compilation of weak-method problem solutions. *Psychological Review, 94*(2), 192–210. https://doi.org/10.1037/0033-295X.94.2.192

Beck, C., & Kosnik, C. (2002). The importance of the university campus program in preservice teacher education: A Canadian case study. *Journal of Teacher Education, 53*(5), 420–432. https://doi.org/10.1177/002248702237396

Behrmann, L., & Souvignier, E. (2013). The relation between teachers' diagnostic sensitivity, their instructional activities, and their students' achievement gains in Reading. *Zeitschrift für Pädagogische Psychologie, 27*(4), 283–293. https://doi.org/10.1024/1010-0652/a000112

Berkhof, M., van Rijssen, H. J., Schellart, A. J., Anema, J. R., & van der Beek, A. J. (2011). Effective training strategies for teaching communication skills to physicians: An overview of systematic reviews. *Patient Education and Counselling, 84*(2), 152–162. https://doi.org/10.1016/j.pec.2010.06.010

Brueckner, L. J. (1928). Analysis of errors in fractions. *The Elementary School Journal, 28*(10), 760–770.

Fischer, F., Kollar, I., Ufer, S., Sodian, B., Hussmann, H., Pekrun, R., Eberle, J., et al. (2014). Scientific reasoning and argumentation: Advancing an interdisciplinary research agenda in education. *Frontline Learning Research, 5*, 28–45. https://doi.org/10.14786/flr.v2i2.96

Frank, B. (2015). *Presence messen in laborbasierter Forschung mit Mikrowelten: Entwicklung und erste Validierung eines Fragebogens zur Messung von Presence*. Springer. https://doi.org/10.1007/978-3-658-08148-5

Fraser, J. W. (2007). *Preparing America's teachers: A history*. Teachers College.

Gartmeier, M., Bauer, J., Fischer, M. R., Hoppe-Seyler, T., Karsten, G., Kiessling, C., Prenzel, M., et al. (2015). Fostering professional communication skills of future physicians and teachers: Effects of e-learning with video cases and role-play. *Instructional Science, 43*(4), 443–462. https://doi.org/10.1007/s11251-014-9341-6

Grossman, P., Compton, C., Igra, D., Ronfeldt, M., Shahan, E., & Williamson, P. (2009a). Teaching practice: A cross-professional perspective. *The Teachers College Record, 111*(9), 2055–2100. https://doi.org/10.1177/0022487114533800

Grossman, P., Hammerness, K., & McDonald, M. (2009b). Redefining teaching, re-imagining teacher education. *Teachers and Teaching: Theory and Practice, 15*(2), 273–289. https://doi.org/10.1080/13540600902875340

Harr, N., Eichler, A., & Renkl, A. (2014, August 20). Integration pedagogical content knowledge and pedagogical/psychological knowledge in mathematics. *Frontiers in Psychology* 5:24. Retrieved from https://www.ncbi.nlm.nih.gov/pmc/articles/PMC4139073/

Heckmann, K. (2006). *Zum Dezimalbruchverständnis von Schülerinnen und Schülern: Theoretische Analyse und empirische Befunde*. Logos.

Heitzmann, N., Seidel, T., Opitz, A., Hetmanek, A., Wecker, C., Fischer, M., Ufer, S., Schmidmaier, R., Neuhaus, B., Siebeck, M., Stürmer, K., Obersteiner, A., Reiss, K., Girwidz, R., & Fischer, F. (2019). Facilitating diagnostic competences in simulations in higher education. *Frontline Learning Research, 7*(4), 1–24. https://doi.org/10.14786/flr.v7i4.384

Herppich, S., Praetorius, A.-K., Förster, N., Glogger-Frey, I., Karst, K., Leutner, D., Südkamp, A., et al. (2017). Teachers' assessment competence: Integrating knowledge-, process-, and product-oriented approaches into a competence-oriented conceptual model. *Teaching and Teacher Education, 76*, 181–193. https://doi.org/10.1016/j.tate.2017.12.001

Jacobs, V. R., Lamb, L. L. C., & Philipp, R. A. (2010). Professional noticing of children's mathematical thinking. *Journal for Research in Mathematics Education, 41*(2), 169–202.

Kaiser, J., Praetorius, A.-K., Südkamp, A., & Ufer, S. (2017). Die enge Verwobenheit von diagnostischem und pädagogischem Handeln als Herausforderung bei der Erfassung diagnostischer Kompetenz. In A. Südkamp & A.-K. Praetorius (Eds.), *Diagnostische Kompetenz von Lehrkräften—Theoretische und methodische Weiterentwicklungen* (pp. 114–122). Waxmann.

Karst, K., Klug, J., & Ufer, S. (2017). Strukturierung diagnostischer Situationen im inner- und außerunterrichtlichen Handeln von Lehrkräften. In A. Südkamp & A.-K. Praetorius (Eds.), *Diagnostische Kompetenz von Lehrkräften—Theoretische und methodische Weiterentwicklungen* (pp. 95–113). Waxmann.

Kleickmann, T., Richter, D., Kunter, M., & Elsner, J. (2012). Teachers' content knowledge and pedagogical content knowledge: The role of structural differences in teacher education. *Journal of Teacher Education, 64*(1), 90–106. https://doi.org/10.1177/0022487112460398

Klug, J., Bruder, S., Kelava, A., Spiel, C., & Schmitz, B. (2013). Diagnostic competence of teachers. A process model that accounts for diagnosing learning behavior tested by means of a case scenario. *Teaching and Teacher Education, 30*, 38–46. https://doi.org/10.1016/j.tate.2012.10.004

KMK. (2004). *Standards für die Lehrerbildung*. Bildungswissenschaften, Bericht der Arbeitsgruppe.

Lane, C., & Rollnick, S. (2007). The use of simulated patients and role-play in communication skills training: A review of the literature to august 2005. *Patient Education and Counseling, 67*(1), 13–20. https://doi.org/10.1016/j.pec.2007.02.011

Lane, C., Hood, K., & Rollnick, S. (2008). Teaching motivational interviewing: Using role play is as effective as using simulated patients. *Medical Education, 42*(6), 637–644. https://doi.org/10.1111/j.1365-2923.2007.02990.x

Lortie-Forgues, H., Tian, J., & Siegler, R. (2015). Why is learning fraction and decimal arithmetic so difficult? *Developmental Review, 38*, 201–221. https://doi.org/10.1016/j.dr.2015.07.008

Mamede, S., van Gog, T., Moura, A. S., de Faria, R. M. D., Peixoto, J. M., Rikers, R. M. J. P., & Schmidt, H. G. (2012). Reflection as a strategy to foster medical students' acquisition of diagnostic competence. *Medical Education, 46*, 464–472. https://doi.org/10.1111/j.1365-2923.2012.04217.x

Mamede, S., van Gog, T., Sampaio, A. M., de Faria, R. M. D., Maria, J. D., & Schmidt, H. G. (2014). How can students' diagnostic competence benefit most from practice with clinical cases? The effects of structured reflection on future diagnosis of the same and novel diseases. *Academic Medicine, 89*(1), 121–127. https://doi.org/10.1097/ACM.0000000000000076

McDonough, A., Clarke, B., & Clarke, D. M. (2002). Understanding, assessing and developing children's mathematical thinking: The power of a one-to-one interview for preservice teachers in providing insights into appropriate pedagogical practices. *International Journal of Educational Research, 37*(2), 211–226. https://doi.org/10.1016/S0883-0355(02)00061-7

Ministry of Education. (2008). *Teaching fractions, decimals, and percentages*. Ministry of Education.

Nickerson, S. D., Lamb, L., & LaRochelle, R. (2017). Challenges in measuring secondary mathematics teachers' professional noticing of students' mathematical thinking. In E. Schack, M. Fisher, & J. Wilhelm (Eds.), *Teacher noticing: Bridging and broadening perspectives, contexts, and frameworks. Research in mathematics education* (pp. 381–398). Springer. https://doi.org/10.1007/978-3-319-46753-5_22

Padberg, F., & Wartha, S. (2017). *Didaktik der Bruchrechnung*. Springer Spektrum. https://doi.org/10.1007/978-3-662-52969-0

Schack, E. O., Fisher, M. H., Thomas, J. N., Eisenhardt, S., Tassell, J., & Yoder, M. (2013). Prospective elementary school teachers' professional noticing of children's early numeracy. *Journal of Mathematics Teacher Education, 16*(5), 379–397. https://doi.org/10.1007/s10857-013-9240-9

Schrader, F.-W. (2013). Diagnostische Kompetenz von Lehrpersonen. *Beiträge zur Lehrerinnen- und Lehrerbildung, 31*(2), 154–165.
Schubert, T., Friedmann, F., & Regenbrecht, H. (2001). The experience of presence: Factor analytic insights. *Presence, 10*(3), 266–281.
Seidel, T., & Stürmer, K. (2014). Modeling and measuring the structure of professional vision in preservice teachers. *American Educational Research Journal, 51*(4), 739–771. https://doi.org/10.3102/0002831214531321
Seidel, T., Blomberg, G., & Stürmer, K. (2010). OBSERVE—Validierung eines videobasierten Instruments zur Erfassung der professionellen Wahrnehmung von Unterricht. In E. Klieme, D. Leutner, & M. Kenk (Eds.), *Kompetenzmodellierung. Zwischenbilanz des DFG-Schwerpunktprogramms und Perspektiven des Forschungsansatzes. 56. Beiheft der Zeitschrift für Pädagogik* (pp. 296–306). Beltz.
Seidel, T., Stürmer, K., Schäfer, S., & Jahn, G. (2015). How preservice teachers perform in teaching events regarding generic teaching and learning components. *Zeitschrift für Entwicklungspsychologie und Pädagogische Psychologie, 47*(2), 84–96. https://doi.org/10.1026/0049-8637/a000125
Shavelson, R. J. (2012). Assessing business-planning competence using the collegiate learning assessment as a prototype. *Empirical Research in Vocational Education and Training, 4*(1), 77–90.
Spinath, B. (2005). Akkuratheit der Einschätzung von Schülermerkmalen durch Lehrer und das Konstrukt der diagnostischen Kompetenz. *Zeitschrift für Pädagogische Psychologie, 19*, 85–95. https://doi.org/10.1024/1010-0652.19.12.85
Stegmann, K., Pilz, F., Siebeck, M., & Fischer, F. (2012). Vicarious learning during simulations: Is it more effective than hands-on training? *Medical Education, 46*(10), 1001–1008. https://doi.org/10.1111/j.1365-2923.2012.04344.x
Steinle, V. (2004). *Changes with age in students' misconceptions of decimal numbers (unpublished doctoral dissertation)*. Department of Science and Mathematics Education, The University of Melbourne.
Thiede, K., Brendefur, J., Carney, M., Champion, J., Turner, L., Stewart, R., & Osguthorpe, R. (2018). Improving the accuracy of teachers' judgments of student learning. *Teaching and Teacher Education, 76*, 106–115. https://doi.org/10.1016/j.tate.2018.08.004
van den Kieboom, L. A., Magiera, M. T., & Moyer, J. C. (2014). Exploring the relationship between K-8 prospective teachers' algebraic thinking proficiency and the questions they pose during diagnostic algebraic thinking interviews. *Journal of Mathematics Teacher Education, 17*(5), 429–461. https://doi.org/10.1007/s10857-013-9264-1
van Es, E., & Sherin, M. G. (2002). Learning to notice: Scaffolding new teachers' interpretations of classroom interactions. *Journal of Technology and Teacher Education, 10*(4), 571–596.
Weinert, F.-E. (2001). Concept of competence: A conceptual clarification. In D. S. Rychen & L. H. Salganik (Eds.), *Defining and selecting key competences* (pp. 45–65). Hogrefe & Huber.

Open Access This chapter is licensed under the terms of the Creative Commons Attribution 4.0 International License (http://creativecommons.org/licenses/by/4.0/), which permits use, sharing, adaptation, distribution and reproduction in any medium or format, as long as you give appropriate credit to the original author(s) and the source, provide a link to the Creative Commons license and indicate if changes were made.

The images or other third party material in this chapter are included in the chapter's Creative Commons license, unless indicated otherwise in a credit line to the material. If material is not included in the chapter's Creative Commons license and your intended use is not permitted by statutory regulation or exceeds the permitted use, you will need to obtain permission directly from the copyright holder.

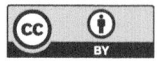

Chapter 6
Diagnosing the Instructional Quality of Biology Lessons Based on Staged Videos: Developing DiKoBi, A Video-Based Simulation

Maria Kramer, Julia Stürmer, Christian Förtsch, Tina Seidel, Stefan Ufer, Martin R. Fischer, and Birgit J. Neuhaus

This chapter's simulation at a glance

Domain	Teacher education
Topic	Diagnosing subject-specific challenging situations in biology instruction
Learner's task	Identifying and describing biology-specific challenges in instruction, reasoning about them by linking their description to scientific theories, and proposing alternative teaching strategies
Target group	Pre-service biology teachers in various stages of their studies and early career practitioners
Diagnostic mode	Individual diagnosing
Sources of information	Interaction; observation of videotaped classroom situations showing the behavior of a teacher and students
Special features	Using the video-based simulation as an assessment and learning tool; use of the simulation links to the model of professional vision

M. Kramer (✉) · J. Stürmer · C. Förtsch · B. J. Neuhaus
Biology Education, Faculty for Biology, LMU Munich, Munich, Germany
e-mail: maria.kramer@biologie.uni-muenchen.de; didaktik.biologie@lrz.uni-muenchen.de

T. Seidel
Friedl Schöller Endowed Chair for Educational Psychology, School of Education, Technical University of Munich (TUM), Munich, Germany

S. Ufer
Chair of Mathematics Education, LMU Munich, Munich, Germany

M. R. Fischer
Institute for Medical Education, University Hospital, LMU Munich, Munich, Germany

© The Author(s) 2022
F. Fischer, A. Opitz (eds.), *Learning to Diagnose with Simulations*,
https://doi.org/10.1007/978-3-030-89147-3_6

6.1 Diagnosing in the Teaching Context

Teachers need to create domain-specific learning activities in the classroom, as these activities strongly influence students' learning (Seidel & Shavelson, 2007). Thus, professional knowledge about implementing these activities is a necessary prerequisite for teachers' performance in the classroom, and thus also for instructional quality (Förtsch et al., 2016, 2018b; Seidel & Shavelson, 2007). University education should not only offer opportunities for pre-service teachers to gain professional knowledge in setting up these activities, but should also support pre-service teachers in applying their knowledge and developing their competences in assessing learning situations during actual teaching (Grossman & McDonald, 2008). Assessing learning situations also means providing on-the-fly diagnoses (Shavelson et al., 2008). As mentioned in the introduction by Fischer et al. (2022), diagnosing describes the "process of goal-oriented collection and integration of case-specific information to reduce uncertainty in order to make [...] educational decisions" (Heitzmann et al., 2019). These educational decisions aim at achieving effective teaching that exhibits the characteristics of instructional quality within a given subject. For successful diagnosis of teaching and learning, an evidence-based approach seems to be a promising way to develop diagnostic competences (Helmke & Lenske, 2013). Following Blömeke et al. (2015), diagnostic competences can be modeled as a continuum that encompassing dispositions, such as professional knowledge; situation-specific skills, such as noticing and reasoning; and an observable performance or an output, such as the quality of diagnostic results. The diagnostic results can be assessed in terms of both the accuracy and efficiency of the diagnosis (Südkamp & Praetorius, 2017). Teachers' noticing of challenging classroom situations and their reasoning about them can vary depending on their professional knowledge (Seidel & Stürmer, 2014; van Es & Sherin, 2002). However, the execution of situation-specific skills during the diagnostic process eventually determines teachers' performance in the classroom (Blömeke et al., 2015). In turn, teaching performance also influences teachers' professional knowledge and situation-specific skills while planning, teaching, and reflecting upon instruction (Santagata & Yeh, 2016; Hume et al., 2019). Thus, we assume bidirectionality for the development of diagnostic competences as well. In addition, researchers have emphasized that practical experience can positively affect teachers' professional development and thus also their development of diagnostic competences (Stahnke et al., 2016).

Therefore, teacher education should find ways to foster pre-service teachers' acquisition of professional knowledge and situation-specific skills as part of teachers' diagnostic competences. Video-based simulations such as DiKoBi (German acronym for "diagnostic competences of biology teachers in biology classrooms") are one way to foster diagnostic competences to assess learning situations.

6.2 Theoretical Background

The following sections specify professional knowledge, situation-specific skills, and teachers' performance as indicators of teachers' diagnostic competences. Furthermore, ways of scaffolding these competences are outlined.

6.2.1 Teachers' Professional Knowledge

Based on the work of Shulman (1987), teachers' professional knowledge can be divided into three facets: content knowledge (CK), pedagogical content knowledge (PCK), and pedagogical knowledge (PK) (cf. Baumert & Kunter, 2013; Blömeke et al., 2010; Förtsch et al., 2018a). According to these conceptualizations, teachers need to use all three knowledge facets when teaching in the classroom. More teaching experience often comes along with more organized and integrated knowledge structures about teaching (de Jong & Ferguson-Hessler, 1996). De Jong and Ferguson-Hessler recognized that in-service teachers' domain-specific knowledge schemas can be described as organized and structured, whereas the pre-service teachers' knowledge base is characterized by superficial elements and missing links to fundamental principles relevant to the domain. Furthermore, research shows a positive relation between teachers' professional knowledge and expertise, on the one hand, and instructional quality on the other (Hill et al., 2007; Blömeke et al., 2010). Borko (2004) emphasized that in-service teachers can recall their knowledge and teaching strategies in varying situations in the classroom. Thus, to develop professional knowledge that is applicable and transferable in various teaching situations, pre-service teachers need opportunities to put their knowledge into practice (Darling-Hammond, 2010). Observing and evaluating teaching situations with regard to instructional quality can be seen as one step toward this practice. Observing teaching situations can call up teachers' knowledge and help them enhance their situation-specific cognitive structures by remembering and adapting solutions. Over time, this process leads to growing expertise (Kolodner, 1992; Prawat, 1989).

However, research is still needed to examine how professional knowledge influences diagnostic competences and how the acquisition of these competences can be fostered. Furthermore, previous research has pointed out that different routes for the acquisition of professional knowledge exist. Kleickmann et al. (2017) note that in the sequence of addressing each knowledge facet (CK, PCK, and PK) within the process of knowledge acquisition is important. However, further research is needed to investigate the effects of different ways of fostering professional knowledge on diagnostic competences.

6.2.2 Situation-Specific Skills for Diagnosing

Situation-specific skills are an important mediator between teachers' dispositions and their performance. When observing classroom situations, teachers use situation-specific skills to diagnose the situation and derive an appropriate teaching action resulting from their diagnosis (Borko et al., 2008). Though different conceptualizations of situation-specific skills exist, they all describe aspects of reasoning processes. Within teacher education, different conceptualizations for describing teachers' professional competences have already been compared and used to complement understanding of teachers' competences (Santagata & Yeh, 2016; Blömeke & Kaiser, 2017). Whereas previous research solely focused on teachers' individual characteristics, the complementary frameworks also considered situational and social dependencies of teachers' development of professional competences (Blömeke et al., 2015). However, an interdisciplinary comparison has not yet been conducted, even though researchers have emphasized that comparing and combining conceptualizations of reasoning and argumentation might bring benefits for science education and thus for science teacher education as well (Bricker & Bell, 2008). In this vein, O'Donnell and Levin (2001) described an increasing number of perspectives and principles from psychology that have been adopted in education. We focus on comparing two representative situation-specific skills that are relevant in the context of diagnosing—one commonly used in teacher education and one commonly used in psychology (see Table 6.1). Furthermore, these two representative skills are considered as relevant representations of models used across the different projects included in this volume. Thus, we expect clarification in terms of greater understanding across the interdisciplinary projects as well.

Researchers on teachers' expertise describe professional vision as an important situation-specific skill to improve instructional quality (Stürmer & Seidel, 2015; Kersting et al., 2012; Goodwin, 1994). Professional vision includes the ability to notice classroom events that are relevant for students' learning as well as the ability to reason about these events (Seidel & Stürmer, 2014; van Es & Sherin, 2002). When teachers reason about noteworthy classroom events, three reasoning skills are crucial: *description, explanation,* and *prediction. Description* is conceptualized as teachers stating "relevant aspects of a noticed teaching situation and learning

Table 6.1 Systematizing situation-specific skills for diagnosing classroom situations

Situation-specific skills for diagnosing (Blömeke et al., 2015)	
Professional vision (Seidel & Stürmer, 2014)	Diagnostic activities (Heitzmann et al., 2019)

• Noticing
• Reasoning
  – Description
  – Explanation
  – Prediction
	• Identifying problems
	• Generating evidence
	• Evaluating evidence
	• Drawing conclusions

The conceptualizations of professional vision and diagnostic activities are itemized based on Blömeke et al.'s (2015) situation-specific skills components without making further judgements" (Seidel & Stürmer, 2014, p. 745). *Explanation* includes teachers' use of knowledge to reason about the noticed aspects by linking them to concepts and theories; and *prediction* is described as teachers deriving consequences from "observed events in terms of student learning" (Seidel & Stürmer, 2014, p. 746). Additionally, rectifications can be made. These situation-specific skills are considered crucial for professionally observing and interpreting classroom situations and thus also for teachers' performance in the classroom (Borko, 2004; Blömeke et al., 2015).

Epistemic activities can be considered another conceptualization of reasoning skills, which describe activities during reasoning and argumentation (Heitzmann, 2013; Fischer et al., 2014). In the context of diagnostic processes, these activities are called diagnostic activities and are required for generating knowledge (Heitzmann et al., 2019; Chernikova et al., 2022). When diagnosing classroom situations, teachers do not necessarily execute all diagnostic activities. We assume that *identifying problems, generating evidence, evaluating evidence,* and *drawing conclusions* are of particular interest when diagnosing the classroom situations in DiKoBi. *Identifying problems* occurs when teachers identify a problematic event within a classroom situation. For *generating evidence,* different approaches exist: Either evidence can be generated in a hypothetico-deductive approach with an experimental design or in an inductive approach. The inductive approach might be particularly relevant with regard to the diagnosis of classroom situations. Here, problematic events are observed, compared, and described in a purposeful way. *Evaluating evidence* occurs when teachers assess their observed and described evidence regarding its support for a claim or theory. *Drawing conclusions* occurs when teachers make predictions concerning students' learning or suggest an alternative teaching action. When assigning these activities to the conceptualization of professional vision, *identifying problems* corresponds to *noticing, generating evidence* corresponds to *description,* and *drawing conclusions* corresponds to *prediction.* From a theoretical perspective, *evidence evaluation* might be assigned to *explanation.* However, the two do not describe exactly the same construct and thus do not overlap completely. *Explanation* is considered to link a theory to generated evidence, which might be one facet of *evidence evaluation* (Kramer et al., 2021).

Even though both conceptualizations, professional vision and diagnostic activities, contain situation-specific skills in the context of reasoning, it is not clear as to what degree the two conceptualizations agree with one another and whether combining them to describe diagnostic processes has added value.

6.2.3 Instructional Quality in Biology Lessons

Depending on teachers' professional knowledge and situation-specific skills, teachers make pedagogical decisions that at least partially become visible as teaching performance in the classroom (Blömeke et al., 2015). This performance is crucial for teaching effectiveness and thus for instructional quality (Kyriakides et al., 2013).

Research has identified general features as well as subject-specific features of instructional quality (Wüsten, 2010). General features are classroom management, supportive climate, and cognitive activation (Baumert et al., 2010; Lipowsky et al., 2009). Classroom management and supportive climate are assumed to act as prerequisites for the implementation of subject-specific features (Dorfner et al., 2018b). Cognitive activation requires the specific subject to be taken into account (Förtsch et al., 2017). To achieve this subject specificity, Wüsten (2010) compiled a classification of biology-specific features that are important for instructional quality in biology lessons. These include content structuring of the lesson, complexity of tasks, cumulative learning, use of technical language, dealing with students' errors and feedback, use of models, use of experiments, and scientific working methods. Research has shown that the clarity of goals had positive effects on students' learning and motivation (Seidel et al., 2005b). Also, an error-tolerant classroom culture showed positive effects on the affective level (Rach et al., 2013). Furthermore, knowledge linking as part of cumulative learning turned out to foster students' knowledge structure (Wadouh et al., 2014). By teaching interrelated facts and concepts instead of isolated facts, students were cognitively activated. Cognitive activation is considered to be a key feature of instructional quality in biology lessons and is associated with several of the above-mentioned features of instructional quality (Dorfner et al., 2018b; Förtsch et al., 2017). Cognitive activation can be influenced via tasks that promote students' cognitive engagement (Chi & Wylie, 2014). Additionally, students' learning can be fostered by a sophisticated use of models that increases scientific reasoning skills (Förtsch et al., 2018b). Scientific reasoning is also important when solving problems in biology (Dorfner et al., 2018a; Mayer, 2007). When using experiments, embedding them in everyday life contexts is a predictor for instructional quality (Tesch & Duit, 2004). The implementation of process variables during experiments can be seen as part of this embedding, which fosters scientific reasoning (Mayer, 2007). Teachers might also have to reconsider their use of professional terms in biology lessons. Dorfner et al. (2019) emphasized that using a high number of professional terms negatively affects students' learning and interest.

To summarize, much effort has been made in research on instructional quality features to identify subject-specific features and foster teachers' knowledge about these features that greatly influence students' learning (Seidel & Shavelson, 2007). Therefore, fostering teachers' subject-specific knowledge is vitally important in terms of effective teaching and its evaluation.

6.2.4 Scaffolds for Facilitating Diagnostic Competences

When seeking to establish instructional quality, diagnostic competences (professional knowledge, situation-specific skills, and performance) are a crucial part of teachers' expertise (Blömeke et al., 2015). Hence, situations that foster the acquisition of diagnostic competences, and thus the transfer of professional knowledge to practice, are needed (Heitzmann, 2013). These situations can be provided by video-based instruments such as simulations (Seidel & Stürmer, 2014). To support teachers in applying their knowledge when diagnosing classroom situations, scaffolds can be used. Scaffolds can be seen as an adaptive support for teachers in carrying out tasks or trying to achieve certain goals (Quintana et al., 2004).

One approach to fostering the acquisition and application of professional knowledge is the use of prompts during the solution of the task as a scaffolding option. Prompts can be content-related and thus support novice teachers in activating relevant knowledge structures and linking them to the teaching situation by referring to specific information; or they can provide strategic hints on how to effectively execute diagnostic activities (cf. Wildgans-Lang et al., 2022; Hannafin et al., 1999; Seidel & Stürmer, 2014). Thus, teachers can develop new connections between their knowledge structures and their classroom performance. Research on the teaching of foreign languages has shown that video-based simulations can foster teachers' application of PK and PCK to their own classroom teaching under certain conditions. The effect occurred only if pre-service teachers were supported by hints from the video-based simulations shown to them before they interacted with a simulation (Goeze et al., 2014). Since the effects of different types of prompts and their embedding in simulations have not yet been investigated, further systematic studies are necessary.

6.3 Research Questions and Objectives

As there is hardly any research measuring teachers' diagnostic competences in light of contextualized and situated real-world biology demands (Blömeke et al., 2015), this project investigated pre-service teachers diagnosing real classroom situations in the context of a video-based simulation named DiKoBi. The situations are focused on the whole class to give participants the opportunity to apply their diagnostic competences with a subject-specific view under conditions similar to real classrooms. More precisely, we want to investigate the relation between professional knowledge; the use of situation-specific skills, which are operationalized as diagnostic activities and professional vision; and the quality of the diagnostic results. Within this project, we focus on the facilitation of professional knowledge as part of diagnostic competences, and its influence on the execution of situation-specific skills and the accuracy and efficiency of the diagnostic results. Additionally, the effects of addressing the different knowledge facets in a successive or integrated way during teachers' acquisition of professional knowledge are investigated. We use our developed video-based simulation DiKoBi to measure situation-specific skills, the accuracy and efficiency of the diagnostic results. Furthermore, we want to investigate how diagnostic competences can be fostered with DiKoBi. Therefore, we analyze the influence of scaffolding by using different prompts during the solution of the task. The main research questions of the project are:

1. What is the relation between the different facets of professional knowledge (CK, PCK, and PK) and the use of situation-specific skills as well as the quality of the diagnostic results?
2. What are the effects of addressing CK, PCK, and PK in (a) a successive way or (b) in an integrated way on the acquisition of diagnostic competences?
3. What are the effects of prompting (regarding content or diagnostic activities) during the solution of the tasks in DiKoBi on the acquisition of diagnostic competences among pre-service teachers with different levels of professional knowledge?

6.4 Video-Based Simulation

In this project, the German online learning platform DiKoBi serves as a video-based simulation, in which six classroom situations are embedded. The classroom situations represent challenging dimensions in biology classrooms: (1) students' level of cognitive activities (Förtsch et al., 2016), (2) dealing with students' ideas and errors (Rach et al., 2013), (3) use of technical language (Dorfner et al., 2019; Wüsten, 2010), (4) use of experiments (Mayer, 2007), (5) use of models (Förtsch et al., 2018b; Werner et al., 2017), and (6) conceptual understanding (Förtsch et al., 2017). Pre-service teachers had to diagnose effective teaching using DiKoBi. To represent a real-world context, the classroom situation for diagnosis focuses on interactions between a teacher and a whole class, not a single student. Thus, the diagnostic situation is individual and based on (observed) interaction (Chernikova et al., 2022).

To show specific classroom situations, staged videos were recorded and embedded in the learning platform. The use of staged videos is considered an appropriate method for analyzing the complex situations of classroom teaching and learning as well as measuring teachers' expertise in such classroom situations, where teacher knowledge is activated by the real-life context (Hoth et al., 2018; Kersting et al., 2010; Stürmer & Seidel, 2015).

6.4.1 Development of Staged Videos

We scripted three consecutive lessons on the topic of 'skin' to be videotaped, focusing on three different subtopics. By doing this, we were able to vary the lesson shown in the videos in case participants use DiKoBi more than once. Instruction on the subtopics was guided by standards from the Bavarian curriculum on the content area 'senses and sensory organs' (State Institute of School Quality and Educational Research Munich, 2018). The first lesson focuses on the subtopic "skin as a sensory organ" in Grade 5, the second lesson on the subtopic "protective functions of the skin," and the third lesson on the subtopic "regulation of body temperature." Each lesson was divided into six cases, each focusing on a different instructional quality feature of biology lessons.

For each of the six dimensions of instructional quality, we videotaped lessons on three different quality levels based on scripts. For each case, there is a basic version showing a part of the lesson in which relevant features of the dimension of instructional quality under study are missing. Additionally, there are two other versions showing alternative teaching strategies considering the relevant instructional quality features. To ensure the comparability of the three video versions, the content of the lessons shown in the video for each instructional quality feature is identical. We ultimately prepared 18 simulated video cases for each of the three lessons.

The staged video cases were videotaped in school afternoon workshops at a secondary school in Bavaria (for a more detailed description, see Kramer et al., 2020). The workshop took place in a science classroom, which was equipped with cameras for videotaping lessons. The teacher and all speaking students used microphones to improve the sound quality. The workshop program included time for textbook learning, practicing, and video recording.

6.4.2 Use of Simulation and Diagnostic Process

The diagnostic process was measured with three different tasks that require situation-specific skills for diagnosing. First, participants have to watch the video and identify challenging aspects of the classroom situation by noting them down in open text fields in the simulation on the computer (for Task *Describe*, see Fig. 6.1). Second, participants are asked to reason about their described aspects by linking them to subject-related pedagogical theories and concepts (Task *Explain*). Additionally, they have to estimate their confidence about their reflections on the classroom situation by adjusting a slider on a questionnaire scale (from completely unconfident to very confident). Third, participants have to propose an alternative teaching strategy and explain why their selected strategy would improve the classroom situation (Task *Alternative Strategy*). Again, for each classroom situation, participants have to estimate how confident they feel about their described and explained alternative teaching strategy (see Fig. 6.2).

Last, the learning environment DiKoBi can be extended depending on the aim of measurement. In the extended version, participants watch two videos showing teaching alternatives at the end of each of the six different classroom situations, and they are asked to decide which alternative is better from their perspective. In addition, they have to explain using their professional knowledge why they chose the selected alternative. However, a reduced version without video alternatives can be used to measure diagnostic competences. The extended version showing the teaching alternatives can be used to propose ways to optimize the presented classroom situation.

Diagnostic accuracy is determined based on the participants' answers from the text fields, which are assessed with a coding scheme. The coding scheme is theory-

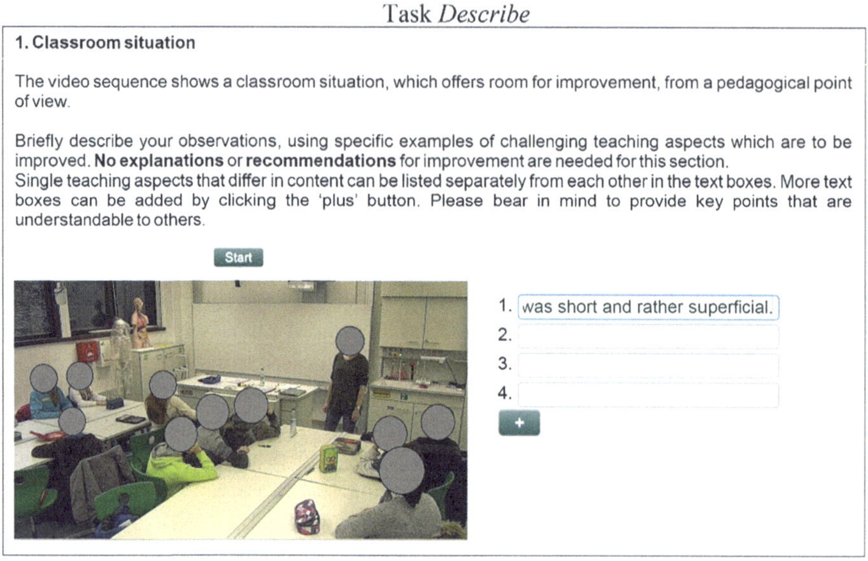

Task *Describe*

1. Classroom situation

The video sequence shows a classroom situation, which offers room for improvement, from a pedagogical point of view.

Briefly describe your observations, using specific examples of challenging teaching aspects which are to be improved. **No explanations** or **recommendations** for improvement are needed for this section.
Single teaching aspects that differ in content can be listed separately from each other in the text boxes. More text boxes can be added by clicking the 'plus' button. Please bear in mind to provide key points that are understandable to others.

1. was short and rather superficial.
2.
3.
4.

Fig. 6.1 Design of the first task. Participants are asked to note identified challenging teaching aspects in the open text fields on the right

based and includes references to biology-specific features of instructional quality, to which participants have to refer during the diagnostic processes. Diagnostic efficiency can be determined based on the participants' time spent completing the tasks in relation to accuracy. The coding scheme also includes descriptions for coding the participants' diagnostic competences based on their conceptualizations of professional vision and diagnostic activities.

6.4.3 Generating Data with DiKoBi

In the following example, the process of data generation to measure situation-specific skills in the context of diagnosing instructional quality is elaborated for a teacher named Paul, illustratively shown for the Task *Describe* and the Task *Alternative Strategy* with reference to diagnosing the first classroom situation in DiKoBi. The assigned tasks guide the diagnostic process and therefore the execution of situation-specific skills.

Table 6.2 presents Paul's answers as well as the corresponding codings and their operationalization within the different conceptualizations. After watching the video of the first classroom situation, the Task *Describe* asks for a description of challenging aspects of the watched classroom situation. To answer the Task *Describe*, Paul has to generate information by describing the problem he has identified in the classroom situation. Paul's note *(The introduction was short and rather superficial)*

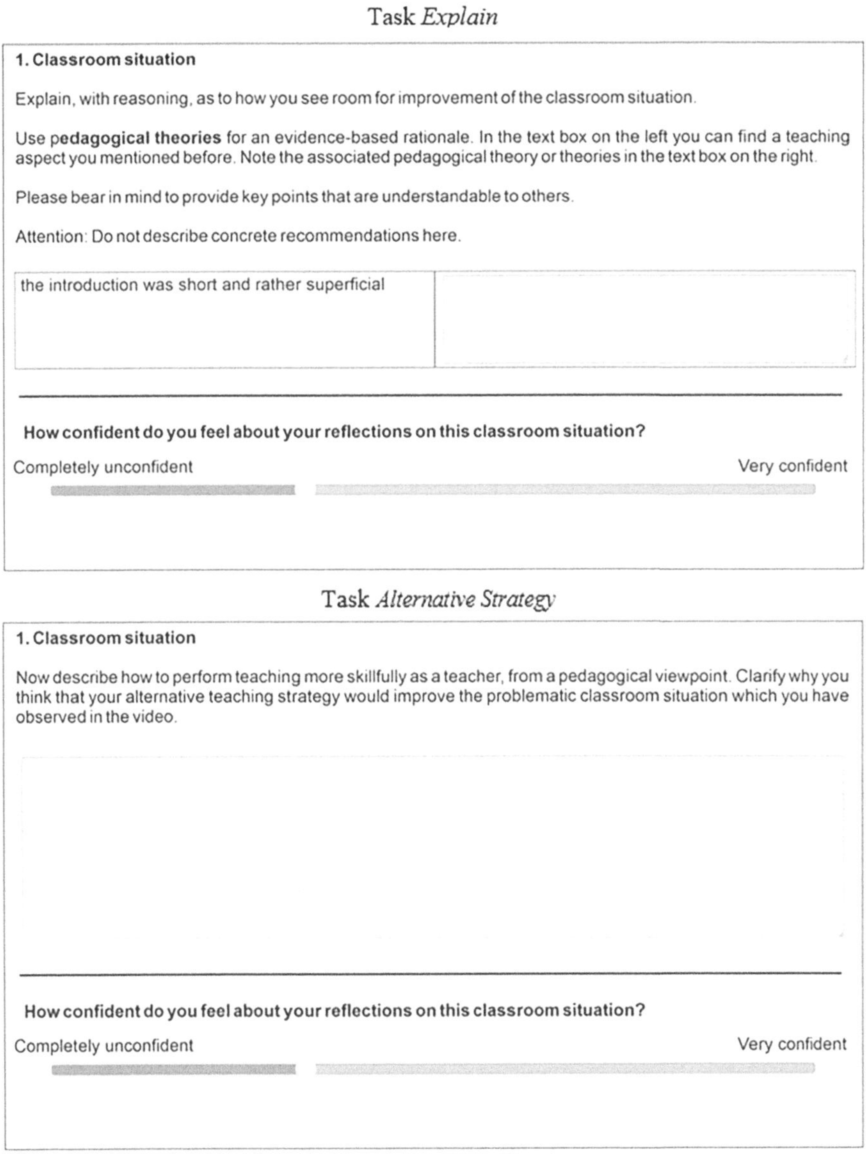

6 Diagnosing the Instructional Quality of Biology Lessons Based on Staged...

Task *Explain*

1. Classroom situation

Explain, with reasoning, as to how you see room for improvement of the classroom situation.

Use **pedagogical theories** for an evidence-based rationale. In the text box on the left you can find a teaching aspect you mentioned before. Note the associated pedagogical theory or theories in the text box on the right.

Please bear in mind to provide key points that are understandable to others.

Attention: Do not describe concrete recommendations here.

the introduction was short and rather superficial	

How confident do you feel about your reflections on this classroom situation?

Completely unconfident   Very confident

Task *Alternative Strategy*

1. Classroom situation

Now describe how to perform teaching more skillfully as a teacher, from a pedagogical viewpoint. Clarify why you think that your alternative teaching strategy would improve the problematic classroom situation which you have observed in the video.

How confident do you feel about your reflections on this classroom situation?

Completely unconfident   Very confident

Fig. 6.2 Design of Task *Explain* and Task *Alternative Strategy*. Participants are asked for pedagogical rationales as well as alternative teaching strategies. Additionally, participants have to estimate their confidence about the answers they have given

Table 6.2 Part of the coding scheme used for generating data with DiKoBi

Teacher Paul's answers	Situation-specific skills for diagnosing	
	Diagnostic activities (Fischer et al., 2014; Heitzmann et al., 2019)	Professional vision (Seidel & Stürmer, 2014; van Es & Sherin, 2002)
Task *Describe*: Briefly describe your observations... *The introduction was short and rather superficial*	*Generating evidence* Means: Challenging events are observed, compared and described purposively	*Description* Means: Relevant events that influence instructional quality and thus students' learning are listed
Task *Alternative strategy*: Describe how to perform teaching more skillfully... *The teacher could compare the skin and its tasks with a jacket and its tasks. By doing so, he can extrapolate functions of the skin from its structures and features to conclude that functional aspects depend on structural features*	*Drawing conclusions* Means: Consequences that lead to redesign of behavior or environment are derived	*Prediction* Means: Consequences of observed events or alternative teaching strategies are derived

For illustrative purposes, answers from a teacher named Paul are presented and matched with codings from the different conceptualizations

refers to the biology-specific feature "level of students' cognitive activities", which can be enhanced, for example, by reactivating students' prior knowledge. Paul's note shows that he described the observation he made without any further judgments. Thus, he generated evidence for further reasoning. Accordingly, we can code *generating evidence* as the situation-specific skill that occurs using the conceptualization of diagnostic activities. The Task *Alternative Strategy* asks for a description of an alternative teaching strategy to improve on the identified problem. The task targets teachers' ability to conclude how teaching could be performed more skillfully. Paul's answer shows that his alternative strategy supports cognitive activation by comparing structures and functions. Thus, we can code *drawing conclusions* as the situation-specific skill that occurs.

To sum up, by matching teachers' answers with diagnostic activities or aspects of professional vision, we measure situation-specific skills in the process of diagnosing as indicators of diagnostic competences.

6.5 Validation of DiKoBi as a Measurement Instrument

To investigate the validity of DiKoBi for measuring situation-specific skills as part of diagnostic competences, the content and tasks were validated with (a) interviews using think-aloud protocols (Kramer et al., 2020) and (b) expert-novice comparisons. Moreover, the comparability of diagnostic activities and aspects of professional vision as situation-specific skills were examined. Thus, we seek to contribute to clarifying and expanding conceptualizations used in interdisciplinary research fields. (a) Interviews using think-aloud protocols were conducted with five experts who were biology teachers at German secondary schools with an average teaching experience of 9.4 years after teacher training ($SD = 6.9$ years). These experts first watched the six classroom situations to identify challenging teaching aspects. Second, they worked on one classroom situation from DiKoBi by answering the items in the simulation while thinking aloud. Afterwards, their protocols were transcribed and analyzed using qualitative content analysis (Mayring, 2014). Each statement made by the experts in the interviews was matched with one category from professional vision and one from diagnostic activities. The results showed that almost all of our scripted problems were identified in the interviewees' statements, and that the created tasks measure situation-specific skills of the diagnostic process. The results of the comparison of professional vision and diagnostic activities showed that *generating evidence* as a diagnostic activity matched the professional vision aspect *description*, and *drawing conclusions* matched the professional vision aspect *prediction*. The diagnostic activity *evidence evaluation* included explanatory statements, which linked theories and evidence. Additionally, there were evaluative statements that contained a personal assessment of the quality of the generated evidence. The assessment referred to the degree to which the evidence supported the identified challenging classroom situation. The comparison with professional vision showed that explanatory parts of *evidence evaluation* matched the professional vision aspect *explanation* (Kramer et al., 2021). (b) For the expert-novice comparison, 15 in-service teachers with an average teaching experience of 6.1 years ($SD = 5.9$) and 64 pre-service teachers with an average length of study of 2.2 semesters ($SD = 0.7$) worked on DiKoBi. Both experts and novices examined the authenticity of the diagnostic situations presented in the videos. Furthermore, experts' and novices' answers in the open text fields were analyzed for each of the six simulated classroom situations. The described challenges, theoretical rationales, and selected alternatives by experts and novices were compared in terms of the situation-specific skills used. Initial results showed that both experts and novices assessed the videos as authentic. Furthermore, experts used situation-specific skills more extensively.

The above validation results points out that DiKoBi can be used as a valid instrument for measuring diagnostic competences concerning instructional quality. Additionally, we showed that the concepts of professional vision and diagnostic activities contain facets that can be used for conceptual refinement, as we did for the diagnostic activity *evaluating evidence*. Thus, the results promote the understanding of the research projects' fundamental principles based on common discipline-specific theories.

6.6 Interdisciplinary Collaboration

The interdisciplinary collaboration within this project combines expertise on research on teachers' professional competences (e.g., Jüttner & Neuhaus, 2013), video-based teaching (e.g., Seidel et al., 2005a; Seidel & Stürmer, 2014; Ufer & Reiss, 2010), as well as on learning and computer-supported case-based learning in both the mathematical (e.g., Lindmeier, 2011) and medical contexts (e.g., Kopp et al., 2009; Stark et al., 2011). The experiences from this interdisciplinary collaboration enabled us to build the computer-supported video-based simulation DiKoBi, in which different features of instructional quality in biology lessons are presented in the form of staged videos. In accordance with Seidel and Stürmer (2014), who developed a video-based instrument called the Observer Research Tool for measuring professional vision in classroom situations, we developed the biology-specific instrument DiKoBi, which can be used to examine the development of professional vision among pre-service biology teachers. The Observer Research Tool project also investigated which competences teachers need to develop to cope with classroom situations successfully (Koster et al., 2005). The experiences and concepts from the interdisciplinary collaboration can be used to analyze diagnostic competences in a wider approach.

6.7 Conclusion and Possible Applications

This chapter describes the conceptualization, design, and development of the video-based simulation DiKoBi, which focuses on diagnosing effective teaching in terms of instructional quality in the context of biology lessons. A validation study showed that DiKoBi can be used to measure situation-specific skills that are used during diagnostic processes (Kramer et al., 2020). DiKoBi could potentially be used in university courses as a learning environment for professional vision. Additionally, the staged videos from the simulations can be used separately for analyzing teaching examples, discussing features of instructional quality, and linking them to professional terms and concepts. Going forward, we want to contribute to Questions 2 and 4 of the overarching research questions mentioned in the introduction by Fischer et al. (2022) and in the concluding chapter by Opitz et al. (2022). We plan to address the question of how best to support pre-service teachers' learning outcomes by investigating effects of scaffolds such as content-related prompts or prompts focused on diagnostic activities. Furthermore, depending on pre-service teachers' professional knowledge, we want to adapt the scaffolds used in the simulation to better fit learners. Altogether, the developed instrument and its components represent a video-based simulation with the potential to support teachers in transferring professional knowledge to actual decisions in classroom teaching.

Acknowledgments The research presented in this chapter was funded by a grant from the Deutsche Forschungsgemeinschaft (DFG-FOR 2385) to Birgit Neuhaus, Tina Seidel, Stefan Ufer, and Martin R. Fischer (NE 1196/8-1).

References

Baumert, J., & Kunter, M. (2013). The COACTIV model of teachers' professional competence. In M. Kunter, J. Baumert, W. Blum, U. Klusmann, S. Krauss, & M. Neubrand (Eds.), *Cognitive activation in the mathematics classroom and professional competence of teachers. Results from the coactiv project* (pp. 25–48). Springer.

Baumert, J., Kunter, M., Blum, W., Brunner, M., Voss, T., Jordan, A., et al. (2010). Teachers' mathematical knowledge, cognitive activation in the classroom, and student Progress. *American Educational Research Journal, 47*, 133–180. https://doi.org/10.3102/0002831209345157

Blömeke, S., & Kaiser, G. (2017). Understanding the development of teachers' professional competencies as personally, situationally and socially determined. In D. J. Clandinin & J. Husu (Eds.), *International handbook of research on teacher education* (pp. 783–802). Sage.

Blömeke, S., Kaiser, G., & Lehmann, R. (Eds.). (2010). *TEDS-M 2008: Professionelle Kompetenz und Lerngelegenheiten angehender Mathematiklehrkräfte für die Sekundarstufe I im internationalen Vergleich*. Waxmann.

Blömeke, S., Gustafsson, J.-E., & Shavelson, R. J. (2015). Beyond dichotomies. *Zeitschrift für Psychologie, 223*, 3–13. https://doi.org/10.1027/2151-2604/a000194

Borko, H. (2004). Professional development and teacher learning: Mapping the terrain. *Educational Researcher, 33*(8), 3–15.

Borko, H., Roberts, S. A., & Shavelson, R. (2008). Teachers' decision making: From Alan J. bishop to today. In P. Clarkson & N. Presmeg (Eds.), *Critical issues in mathematics education: Major contributions of Alan bishop* (1st ed., pp. 37–67). Springer US.

Bricker, L. A., & Bell, P. (2008). Conceptualizations of argumentation from science studies and the learning sciences and their implications for the practices of science education. *Science Education, 92*, 473–498. https://doi.org/10.1002/sce.20278

Chernikova, O., Heitzmann, N., Opitz, A., Seidel, T., & Fischer, F. (2022). A theoretical framework for fostering diagnostic competences with simulations. In F. Fischer & A. Opitz (Eds.), *Learning to diagnose with simulations—Examples from teacher education and medical education. Springer briefs in education series*. Springer.

Chi, M. T. H., & Wylie, R. (2014). The ICAP framework: Linking cognitive engagement to active learning outcomes. *Educational Psychologist, 49*, 219–243. https://doi.org/10.1080/00461520.2014.965823

Darling-Hammond, L. (2010). Teacher education and the American future. *Journal of Teacher Education, 61*, 35–47. https://doi.org/10.1177/0022487109348024

de Jong, T., & Ferguson-Hessler, M. G. M. (1996). Types and qualities of knowledge. *Educational Psychologist, 31*(2), 105–113.

Dorfner, T., Förtsch, C., Germ, M., & Neuhaus, B. J. (2018a). Biology instruction using a generic framework of scientific reasoning and argumentation. *Teaching and Teacher Education, 75*, 232–243. https://doi.org/10.1016/j.tate.2018.07.003

Dorfner, T., Förtsch, C., & Neuhaus, B. J. (2018b). Effects of three basic dimensions of instructional quality on students' situational interest in sixth-grade biology instruction. *Learning and Instruction, 56*, 42–53. https://doi.org/10.1016/j.learninstruc.2018.03.001

Dorfner, T., Förtsch, C., & Neuhaus, B. J. (2019). Use of technical terms in German biology lessons and its effects on students' conceptual learning. *Research in Science and Technological Education, 38*, 227–251. https://doi.org/10.1080/02635143.2019.1609436

Fischer, F., Kollar, I., Ufer, S., Sodian, B., Hussmann, H., Pekrun, R., et al. (2014). Scientific reasoning and argumentation: Advancing an interdisciplinary research agenda in education. *Frontline Learning Research, 5*, 28–45.

Förtsch, C., Werner, S., von Kotzebue, L., & Neuhaus, B. J. (2016). Effects of biology teachers' professional knowledge and cognitive activation on students' achievement. *International Journal of Science Education, 38*, 2642–2666. https://doi.org/10.1080/09500693.2016.1257170

Förtsch, C., Werner, S., Dorfner, T., von Kotzebue, L., & Neuhaus, B. J. (2017). Effects of cognitive activation in biology lessons on students' situational interest and achievement. *Research in Science Education, 47*, 559–578. https://doi.org/10.1007/s11165-016-9517-y

Förtsch, C., Sommerhoff, D., Fischer, F., Fischer, M., Girwidz, R., Obersteiner, A., et al. (2018a). Systematizing professional knowledge of medical doctors and teachers: Development of an interdisciplinary framework in the context of diagnostic competences. *Educational Sciences, 8*, 207. https://doi.org/10.3390/educsci8040207

Förtsch, S., Förtsch, C., von Kotzebue, L., & Neuhaus, B. (2018b). Effects of teachers' professional knowledge and their use of three-dimensional physical models in biology lessons on students' achievement. *Educational Sciences, 8*, 118. https://doi.org/10.3390/educsci8030118

Goeze, A., Zottmann, J. M., Vogel, F., Fischer, F., & Schrader, J. (2014). Getting immersed in teacher and student perspectives?: Facilitating analytical competence using video cases in teacher education. *Instructional Science, 42*, 91–114. https://doi.org/10.1007/s11251-013-9304-3

Goodwin, C. (1994). Professional vision. *American Anthropologist, 96*(3), 606–633.

Grossman, P., & McDonald, M. (2008). Back to the future: Directions for research in teaching and teacher education. *American Educational Research Journal, 45*, 184–205. https://doi.org/10.3102/0002831207312906

Hannafin, M. J., Land, S. M., & Oliver, K. M. (1999). Open learning environments: Foundations, methods, and models. In C. M. Reigeluth (Ed.), *Instructional-design-theories and models: A new paradigm of instructional theory* (pp. 115–140). Lawrence Erlbaum.

Heitzmann, N. (2013). *Fostering diagnostic competence in different domains. Dissertation.* Ludwig-Maximilians-Universität.

Heitzmann, N., Seidel, T., Opitz, A., Hetmanek, A., Wecker, C., Fischer, M., Ufer, S., Schmidmaier, R., Neuhaus, B., Siebeck, M., Stürmer, K., Obersteiner, A., Reiss, K., Girwidz, R., & Fischer, F. (2019). Facilitating diagnostic competences in simulations in higher education. *Frontline Learning Research, 7*(4), 1–24. https://doi.org/10.14786/flr.v7i4.384

Helmke, A., & Lenske, G. (2013). Unterrichtsdiagnostik als Voraussetzung für Unterrichtsentwicklung. *Beiträge zur Lehrerbildung, 31*(2), 214–233.

Hill, H. C., Ball, D. L., Blunk, M., Goffney, I. M., & Rowan, B. (2007). Validating the ecological assumption: The relationship of measure scores to classroom teaching and student learning. *Measurement: Interdisciplinary Research & Perspective, 5*, 107–118. https://doi.org/10.1080/15366360701487138

Hoth, J., Kaiser, G., Döhrmann, M., König, J., & Blömeke, S. (2018). A situated approach to assess teachers' professional competencies using classroom videos. In O. Buchbinder & S. Kuntze (Eds.), *Mathematics teachers engaging with representations of practice: A dynamically evolving field. ICME-13 Monographs* (pp. 23–45). Springer.

Hume, A., Cooper, R., & Borowski, A. (Eds.). (2019). *Repositioning pedagogical content knowledge in teachers' knowledge for teaching science*. Springer.

Jüttner, M., & Neuhaus, B. J. (2013). Validation of a paper-and-pencil test instrument measuring biology teachers' pedagogical content knowledge by using think-aloud interviews. *Journal of Education and Training Studies, 1*(2), 113–125. https://doi.org/10.11114/jets.v1i2.126

Kersting, N. B., Givvin, K. B., Sotelo, F. L., & Stigler, J. W. (2010). Teachers' analyses of classroom video predict student learning of mathematics: Further explorations of a novel measure of teacher knowledge. *Journal of Teacher Education, 61*, 172–181. https://doi.org/10.1177/0022487109347875

Kersting, N. B., Givvin, K. B., Thompson, B. J., Santagata, R., & Stigler, J. W. (2012). Measuring usable knowledge: Teachers' analyses of mathematics classroom videos predict teaching quality and student learning. *American Educational Research Journal, 49*(3), 568–589.

Kleickmann, T., Tröbst, S., Heinze, A., Bernholt, A., Rink, R., & Kunter, M. (2017). Teacher knowledge experiment: Conditions of the development of pedagogical content knowledge. In D. Leutner, J. Fleischer, J. Grünkorn, & E. Klieme (Eds.), *Competence assessment in education: Research, models and instruments. Methodology of educational measurement and assessment* (Vol. 59, pp. 111–129). Springer International.

Kolodner, J. L. (1992). An introduction to case-based reasoning. *Artificial Intelligence Review, 6*, 3–34. https://doi.org/10.1007/BF00155578

Kopp, V., Stark, R., & Fischer, M. R. (2009). Förderung von Diagnosekompetenz durch fallbasiertes Lernen mit ausgearbeiteten Lösungsbeispielen: Evaluation einer computerbasierten Lernumgebung. *Unterrichtswissenschaft, 37*, 17–34. https://doi.org/10.3262/UW0901017

Koster, B., Brekelmans, M., Korthagen, F., & Wubbels, T. (2005). Quality requirements for teacher educators. *Teaching and Teacher Education, 21*, 157–176. https://doi.org/10.1016/j.tate.2004.12.004

Kramer, M., Förtsch, C., Stürmer, J., Förtsch, S., Seidel, T., & Neuhaus, B. J. (2020). Measuring biology teachers' professional vision: Development and validation of a video-based assessment tool. *Cogent Journal, 7*(1), 1–28. https://doi.org/10.1080/2331186X.2020.1823155

Kramer, M., Förtsch, C., Seidel, T., & Neuhaus, B. J. (2021). Comparing Two Constructs for Describing and Analyzing Teachers' Diagnostic Processes. *Studies in Educational Evaluation, 28*. https://doi.org/10.1016/j.stueduc.2020.100973

Kyriakides, L., Christoforou, C., & Charalambous, C. Y. (2013). What matters for student learning outcomes: A meta-analysis of studies exploring factors of effective teaching. *Teaching and Teacher Education, 36*, 143–152. https://doi.org/10.1016/j.tate.2013.07.010

Lindmeier, A. (2011). *Modeling and measuring knowledge and competencies of teachers: A threefold domain-specific structure model for mathematics (Empirische Studien zur Didaktik der Mathematik)* (Vol. 7). Waxmann.

Lipowsky, F., Rakoczy, K., Pauli, C., Drollinger-Vetter, B., Klieme, E., & Reusser, K. (2009). Quality of geometry instruction and its short-term impact on students' understanding of the Pythagorean theorem. *Learning and Instruction, 19*, 527–537. https://doi.org/10.1016/j.learninstruc.2008.11.001

Mayer, J. (2007). Erkenntnisgewinnung als wissenschaftliches Problemlösen. In D. Krüger & H. Vogt (Eds.), *Theorien in der biologiedidaktischen Forschung: Ein Handbuch für Lehramtsstudenten und Doktoranden* (pp. 177–186). Springer.

Mayring, P. (2014). *Qualitative content analysis: Theoretical foundation, basic procedures and software solution*. Beltz. Retrieved December 18, 2018, from https://www.psychopen.eu/fileadmin/user_upload/books/mayring/ssoar-2014-mayring-Qualitative_content_analysis_theoretical_foundation.pdf

O'Donnell, A., & Levin, J. R. (2001). Educational Psychology's healthy growing pains. *Educational Psychologist, 36*(2), 73–82.

Prawat, R. S. (1989). Promoting access to knowledge, strategy, and disposition in students: A research synthesis. *Review of Educational Research, 59*, 1–41. https://doi.org/10.2307/1170445

Quintana, C., Reiser, B. J., Davis, E. A., Krajcik, J., Fretz, E., Duncan, R. G., et al. (2004). A scaffolding design framework for software to support science inquiry. *Journal of the Learning Sciences, 13*, 337–386. https://doi.org/10.1207/s15327809jls1303_4

Rach, S., Ufer, S., & Heinze, A. (2013). Learning from errors: Effects of teachers' training on students' attitudes towards and their individual use of errors. *Proceedings of the National Academy of Sciences, 8*(1), 21–30.

Santagata, R., & Yeh, C. (2016). The role of perception, interpretation, and decision making in the development of beginning teachers' competence. *ZDM, 48*, 153–165. https://doi.org/10.1007/s11858-015-0737-9

Seidel, T., & Shavelson, R. J. (2007). Teaching effectiveness research in the past decade: The role of theory and research design in disentangling meta-analysis results. *Review of Educational Research, 77*, 454–499. https://doi.org/10.3102/0034654307310317

Seidel, T., & Stürmer, K. (2014). Modeling and measuring the structure of professional vision in preservice teachers. *American Educational Research Journal, 51*, 739–771. https://doi.org/10.3102/0002831214531321

Seidel, T., Prenzel, M., & Kobarg, M. (2005a). *How to run a video study: Technical report of the IPN video study*. Waxmann.

Seidel, T., Rimmele, R., & Prenzel, M. (2005b). Clarity and coherence of lesson goals as a scaffold for student learning. *Learning and Instruction, 15*, 539–556. https://doi.org/10.1016/j.learninstruc.2005.08.004

Shavelson, R. J., Young, D. B., Ayala, C. C., Brandon, P. R., Furtak, E. M., Ruiz-Primo, M. A., et al. (2008). On the impact of curriculum-embedded formative assessment on learning: A collaboration between curriculum and assessment developers. *Applied Measurement in Education, 21*, 295–314. https://doi.org/10.1080/08957340802347647

Shulman, L. S. (1987). Knowledge and teaching: Foundations of the new reform. *Havard Educational Review, 57*, 1–22.

Stahnke, R., Schueler, S., & Roesken-Winter, B. (2016). Teachers' perception, interpretation, and decision-making: A systematic review of empirical mathematics education research. *ZDM, 48*, 1–27. https://doi.org/10.1007/s11858-016-0775-y

Stark, R., Kopp, V., & Fischer, M. R. (2011). Case-based learning with worked examples in complex domains: Two experimental studies in undergraduate medical education. *Learning and Instruction, 21*, 22–33. https://doi.org/10.1016/j.learninstruc.2009.10.001

State Institute of School Quality and Educational Research Munich. (2018). *Lehrplan PLUS*. Retrieved December 12, 2018, from https://www.lehrplanplus.bayern.de/fachlehrplan/gymnasium/5/nt_gym.

Stürmer, K., & Seidel, T. (2015). Assessing professional vision in teacher candidates. *Zeitschrift für Psychologie, 223*, 54–63. https://doi.org/10.1027/2151-2604/a000200

Südkamp, A., & Praetorius, A.-K. (Eds.). (2017). *Diagnostische Kompetenz von Lehrkräften*. Waxmann.

Tesch, M., & Duit, R. (2004). Experimentieren im Physikunterricht – Ergebnisse einer Videostudie. *Zeitschrift für Didaktik der Naturwissenschaften, 10*, 51–69.

Ufer, S., & Reiss, K. (2010). Inhaltsübergreifende und inhaltsbezogene strukturierende Merkmale von Unterricht zum Beweisen in der Geometrie - eine explorative Videostudie. *Unterrichtswissenschaft, 38*, 247–265.

van Es, E., & Sherin, M. (2002). Learning to notice: Scaffolding new teachers' interpretations of classroom interactions. *Journal of Technology and Teacher, 10*(4), 571–596.

Wadouh, J., Liu, N., Sandmann, A., & Neuhaus, B. J. (2014). The effect of knowledge linking levels in biology lessons upon students' knowledge structure. *International Journal of Science and Mathematics Education, 12*, 25–47.

Werner, S., Förtsch, C., Boone, W., von Kotzebue, L., & Neuhaus, B. J. (2017). Investigating how german biology teachers use three-dimensional physical models in classroom instruction: A video study. *Research in Science Education, 1*, 195. https://doi.org/10.1007/s11165-017-9624-4

Wildgans-Lang, A., Scheuerer, S., Obersteiner, A., Fischer, F., & Reiss, C. (2022). Learning to diagnose primary students' mathematical competence levels and misconceptions in document-based simulations. In F. Fischer & A. Opitz (Eds.), *Learning to diagnose with simulations—examples from teacher education and medical education*. Springer.

Wüsten, S. (2010). *Allgemeine und fachspezifische Merkmale der Unterrichtsqualität im Fach Biologie: Eine Video- und Interventionsstudie. Dissertation.* Universität Duisburg-Essen.

Open Access This chapter is licensed under the terms of the Creative Commons Attribution 4.0 International License (http://creativecommons.org/licenses/by/4.0/), which permits use, sharing, adaptation, distribution and reproduction in any medium or format, as long as you give appropriate credit to the original author(s) and the source, provide a link to the Creative Commons license and indicate if changes were made.

The images or other third party material in this chapter are included in the chapter's Creative Commons license, unless indicated otherwise in a credit line to the material. If material is not included in the chapter's Creative Commons license and your intended use is not permitted by statutory regulation or exceeds the permitted use, you will need to obtain permission directly from the copyright holder.

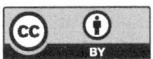

Chapter 7
Learning to Diagnose Secondary School Students' Scientific Reasoning Skills in Physics and Biology: Video-Based Simulations for Pre-Service Teachers

Amadeus J. Pickal, Christof Wecker, Birgit J. Neuhaus, and Raimund Girwidz

This chapter's simulation at a glance

Domain	Teacher education
Topic	Scientific reasoning in physics and biology
Learner's task	To adopt the role of a physics or biology teacher and diagnose—individually or in interdisciplinary collaboration—a student's scientific reasoning skills
Target group	Pre-service teachers
Diagnostic mode	Individual and collaborative diagnosis
Sources of information	(Interactive) videos of pairs of students who perform inquiry activities in physics and biology
Special features	Standardized and parallelized simulations for two different school subjects (physics and biology); possibility to directly interact with the students by "asking" them questions concerning their inquiry activities

A. J. Pickal (✉) · C. Wecker
Institute of Education, University of Hildesheim, Hildesheim, Germany
e-mail: pickal@uni-hildesheim.de

B. J. Neuhaus
Biology Education, Faculty of Biology, LMU Munich, Munich, Germany

R. Girwidz
Chair of Physics Education, LMU Munich, Munich, Germany

© The Author(s) 2022
F. Fischer, A. Opitz (eds.), *Learning to Diagnose with Simulations*,
https://doi.org/10.1007/978-3-030-89147-3_7

7.1 Scientific Reasoning as a Cross-Domain Skill

Many educational objectives in schools refer to subject-specific knowledge and skills, but others refer to cross-curricular or cross-domain skills such as learning strategies, media literacy, or scientific reasoning skills. These skills have in common that they typically cannot be developed without being applied to particular subject-specific content—a so-called *exemplifying domain* (Renkl et al., 2009). For example, a learning strategy such as organizing information by constructing a concept map can only be demonstrated and practiced in the context of a particular topic, such as stem cell research, for example (Hilbert et al., 2008). Fostering scientific reasoning skills requires inquiry tasks concerning phenomena such as factors influencing the image of an object projected through a lens or the growth of plants. Typically, exemplifying domains for the development of cross-domain skills are taken from the body of knowledge contained within school subjects.

Cross-domain skills also have in common that they can be applied to topics from more than one school subject. Learning strategies, media literacy, or—to some degree—scientific reasoning skills can be applied to content from the humanities, the social sciences, or the natural sciences. Therefore, promoting such cross-domain skills can be regarded as a joint task of more than one teacher and more than one school subject (Wecker et al., 2016). Against this backdrop, it may be advisable for teachers of subjects that can serve as exemplifying domains for such cross-domain skills to collaborate in this joint task and share information about individual students' learning progress.

In our own research, we focus on scientific reasoning as a cross-domain skill. Scientific reasoning can be seen as a rather complex set of cognitive activities (Schunn & Anderson, 1999) and is therefore best explained by looking at its subskills. While there are frameworks that differentiate many subskills (Fischer et al., 2014), most researchers distinguish among three dimensions of scientific reasoning skills: (1) formulating hypotheses, (2) designing and conducting experiments, and (3) drawing conclusions from experiments (e.g., de Jong & van Joolingen, 1998; Klahr & Dunbar, 1988). The formulation of hypotheses may be strongly influenced by a person's domain knowledge in a certain field and can be assessed by looking at the specificity of a stated hypothesis (Lazonder et al., 2008). After a hypothesis has been formulated, experiments have to be designed and conducted to test it. At this point, the so-called control of variables strategy, i.e., varying one independent variable from the hypothesis while holding all other variables constant, plays a crucial role in obtaining unequivocal results (Chen & Klahr, 1999; Tschirgi, 1980; Schwichow et al., 2016). Observations from well-designed experiments can then be evaluated and used to draw conclusions about the tested hypothesis. Just as the initial hypothesis, these conclusions again may vary in terms of their specificity. Furthermore, drawing correct inferences about factors that do or do not influence the dependent variable from informative and well-designed comparisons is an important aspect at this point (see Kuhn et al., 1992).

Although there are views that question the existence of cross-domain skills in general or that scientific reasoning in particular is a cross-domain skill (e.g., Tricot & Sweller, 2014; Osborne, 2018), there is research suggesting that there are in fact scientific reasoning skills that can be applied across content areas, at least in related subjects or different scientific subdisciplines (e.g., Kuhn et al., 1992; Schunn & Anderson, 1999). A reason for this ongoing debate about the existence of domain-general or—as we would prefer to call them—cross-domain skills might be different conceptions of the terms "domain" and "domain-general" (Hetmanek et al., 2018), but in light of the strong research tradition on scientific reasoning, we consider scientific reasoning skills as both real and applicable to content from different subjects.

Research from developmental psychology shows that early in the development of a specific subskill of scientific reasoning, it is often applied in one narrow context and no others. Only with time and practice do learners begin to apply the new subskill to a broader range of topics (Kuhn et al., 1992; Zimmerman, 2007) within and across subjects. Hence, the breadth of topics to which a subskill of scientific reasoning can be applied constitutes a quality dimension of the subskill itself. These considerations suggest that practicing scientific reasoning skills in the context of different science subjects such as physics and biology may contribute to the development of higher levels of scientific reasoning skills.

7.1.1 The Role of Teachers' Diagnostic Competences for the Development of Learners' Scientific Reasoning Skills

Teachers' diagnostic competences are an important prerequisite for their adaptive and effective support for their students (Schrader, 2009). Therefore, teachers need to be able to diagnose their students' current skill levels to be able to support them appropriately. The definition by Fischer et al. (2022) is adopted as a basis for the work presented in this chapter.

In order to diagnose correctly, teachers need the cognitive and context-specific performance dispositions to do so (Koeppen et al., 2008). Similar to other cognitive skills, it can be assumed that diagnostic competences are based on teachers' professional knowledge (e.g., Baumert & Kunter, 2006; Förtsch et al., 2018). Therefore, teachers need different types of knowledge (knowing that, knowing how and knowing when and why) as well as content-related facets of knowledge in order to diagnose their students (see Förtsch et al., 2018). Against the background of research on the acquisition of cognitive skills (see VanLehn, 1996), developing diagnostic competences also requires opportunities to apply such knowledge to authentic cases and practice the application of diagnostic competences.

To arrive at a diagnosis, the diagnostician can employ a set of different types of (epistemic) diagnostic activities, including (1) problem identification, (2) questioning, (3) hypothesis generation, (4) construction and redesign of artifacts,

(5) evidence generation, (6) evidence evaluation, (7) drawing conclusions, (8) communication and scrutinizing (see Chernikova et al., 2022; Heitzmann et al., 2019).

While research on diagnostic competences has mainly focused on the accuracy of teachers' judgments of subject-specific knowledge and skills, research on diagnostic competences concerning cross-domain skills, such as scientific reasoning, is still scarce (Südkamp et al., 2012). Therefore, students' scientific reasoning skills were selected as the focus of teachers' diagnostic competences in our present work.

Giving students the chance to conduct scientific experiments in class can create the opportunity to diagnose students' scientific reasoning levels. Two common experiments are experimenting with optical lenses (physics) and experimenting with the growth of plants (biology). The goal while experimenting with plants is to find out which variables (the amount of water, a fertilizer stick, salt and an undefined white powder) influence the growth of a plant (e.g., a bean plant). Therefore, students have to convert their ideas about what influences the growth of a plant into a scientific hypothesis. For example, this could be the idea that the amount of water influences the growth. To test this idea, the students must conduct an experiment. In this case, they would need to vary the quantity of water between two plants to see if there is a difference in growth. Students also need to draw the right conclusions based on the results of the experiment. Based on the growth of the plants, they should be able to determine whether to confirm or reject their hypothesis. The optical lens experiment works quite similarly. Students need to find out which variables (lens curvature, lens size, the distance between the lens and depicted object and an undefined polarizing filter) influence the measurement point at which an object—depicted through an optical lens—appears clear on an imaging screen.

7.1.2 Collaborative Diagnosis of Scientific Reasoning Skills

In the context of daily school routines, diagnosing a student doesn't always have to be a one-person job. Since different teachers experience the same learners in different situations, exchanging information about these learners might be beneficial for teachers to support their students. Still, it is unclear whether interdisciplinary teacher collaboration can help them achieve better results in diagnosing students' scientific reasoning skills. Maybe the information a single teacher can gather in his or her own lessons is already comprehensive enough to be able to arrive at a good diagnosis. However, it is possible that this is not the case and that information from several subjects is needed to be able to get enough information to serve as a basis for a satisfactory diagnosis. This might be especially true when it comes to the question of whether or not a student can apply scientific reasoning skills across school subjects (e.g., physics and biology) in a given domain (science). Therefore, situations in different thematic fields might be necessary to get enough insight (see Kuhn et al., 1992; Zimmerman, 2007). In addition, collaborative diagnosis might have an advantage over the individual development of a diagnosis when the collaborating teachers have different—in the best case complementary—areas of expertise. If this is the case, teachers could benefit from each other by working together (de Wit & Greer, 2008). This idea itself is not new and already very common in different fields of expertise—for example, in the field of medicine. The daily routine in hospitals offers many possibilities or rather necessities for doctors from different fields to work together to improve their chance of arriving at better diagnoses. So-called tumor boards are just one example of such interdisciplinary collaboration. Here, experts from different fields come together to discuss particularly complex malignant diseases. Even though it is also recommended for teachers to collaborate when necessary and to seek help with the management of difficult tasks (Helmke, 2010), this kind of exchange is not institutionalized in the same way. Collaboration is often restricted to a group of teachers teaching the same subject working together to create worksheets or tests. Therefore, there is still a lot of potential for interdisciplinary collaboration, especially when it comes to the need for improving the process of diagnosing students. This approach seems especially promising for teachers from related subjects such as English and German or different scientific subjects. Scientific research also shows that medical students who work in groups arrive at better diagnoses than students working on their own (Hautz et al., 2015). Based on these findings, it seems likely that the same might be true for pre-service teachers. Additionally, it has to be stated that such collaborations can only be fruitful if the process of sharing information is implemented successfully (see Radkowitsch et al., 2022).

7.1.3 Simulations as a Learning Opportunity

Since there are not many opportunities in university-based teacher preparation programs for practicing the diagnosis of scientific reasoning skills in real classroom situations, there is a need for additional training opportunities. In this context, video-based simulations constitute a promising setting for both the training and the measurement of diagnostic competences. Overall, simulations are considered representations of reality segments that offer the possibility to control or manipulate certain parameters (see Chernikova et al., 2022). Simulations can, for example, include videos focusing on specific (classroom) situations and thereby control participants' attention while still creating a realistic scenario. This makes video-based simulations especially interesting for tasks in which learning involves self-regulated exploration—so-called inquiry learning tasks (de Jong, 2006). Another advantage of simulations is that once they are designed and programmed they can be used repeatedly for practice as well as testing.

In contrast to the education of pre-service teachers, learning with simulations is very common in medical education (Peeraer et al., 2007). This is especially interesting since both professions are quite similar when it comes to the need to create training situations for educational purposes. This is the case because in both professions it is difficult to immediately start training in real-life situations. Appropriate alternatives—such as computer-based simulations—can create the opportunity to get this experience.

7.1.4 Video-Based Simulations for Pre-Service Teachers' Diagnosis of Students' Scientific Reasoning Skills

Video-based simulations were developed as an environment to practice and measure pre-service teachers' diagnostic competences concerning students' scientific reasoning skills. As the diagnosis of cross-domain skills such as scientific reasoning skills may benefit from interdisciplinary collaboration, the simulations can be used for individual as well as collaborative diagnosing in interdisciplinary teams made up of teachers of different science subjects.

The simulation can best be understood in terms of the segment of reality it simulates. In this segment of reality, teachers of science subjects (physics or biology) have to diagnose the scientific reasoning skills of individual learners from their classes. For this purpose, they can observe these learners while they perform inquiry tasks in small groups during lessons in their respective subject. Teachers can watch and listen to their students while they generate research questions and formulate hypotheses, design and run experiments and document their observations, and draw conclusions from their observations concerning their hypotheses. They may also interrupt their students by asking questions about their research questions, hypotheses, observations, and conclusions in order to collect information about learners' scientific reasoning that is not directly observable or fully transparent from their activities and dialogue. Based on the information gathered by observing and asking questions of their students during these lessons, they can arrive at a diagnosis of each learner's scientific reasoning skills. Beyond such individual diagnoses, teachers may exchange their observations and discuss their diagnoses with colleagues who teach a different science subject to the same learners and therefore may have collected complementary information about these learners, which may support, contradict, or extend their own diagnoses. Hence, the teachers may collaborate to arrive at a joint diagnosis of each learner's scientific reasoning skills.

The simulation tries to mimic this segment of reality. It is therefore introduced as a kind of role play. Pre-service teachers have to picture themselves as a teacher working in their own school subject. Staged videos of learner dyads are used to simulate a small segment of teachers' experiences during lessons, including the opportunity to observe learners' activities and dialogue and select questions they would like to ask the learners to gain deeper insights into their scientific reasoning during these inquiry tasks. The pre-service teachers' task is to diagnose the scientific reasoning skills of one pre-designated learner from the dyad captured in the video. After watching the video, they are asked to individually write down a diagnosis concerning this learner's scientific reasoning skills. In the collaborative version of

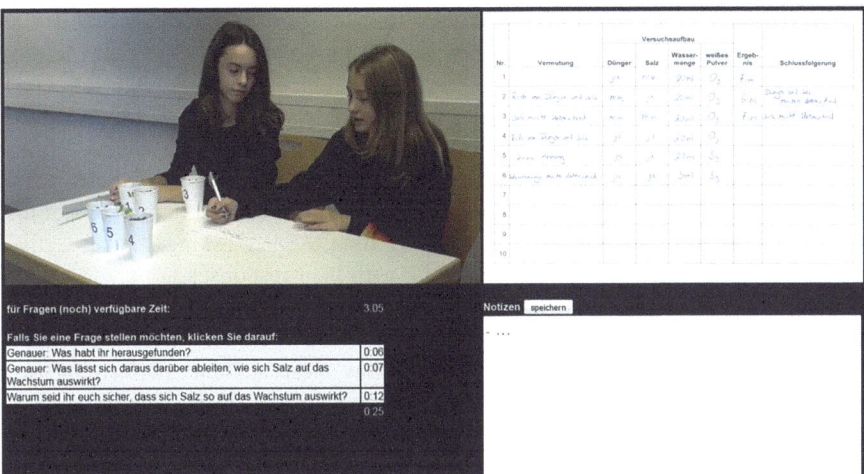

Fig. 7.1 Screenshot of a biology simulation

the simulation, they then enter a phase of interdisciplinary collaboration with a pre-service teacher for the other science subject (physics or biology) in order to generate a joint diagnosis of the learner's scientific reasoning skills that integrates the observations and conclusions from both science subjects. To arrive at their joint diagnosis, they can talk to each other and use material from their individual diagnoses. The video simulations were implemented as follows:

Platform The simulation environment runs in a standard web browser. It is written in PHP, HTML, and Javascript, and uses a MySQL database to store configuration tables and log files. The platform also has test and questionnaire functionalities for empirical studies concerning the instructional design of the video simulations.

Interface During the video simulations with staged videos of learner dyads who collaborate on inquiry tasks, the computer screen is divided into four parts (see Fig. 7.1):

1. The videos are displayed in the top-left area ("video area").
2. The top-right area ("inquiry table") displays a worksheet that the learners in the video use to document their experiments in handwriting. It contains a table with one row per experiment and columns for the research questions and/or hypotheses, the settings of the four independent variables, the measured values of the dependent variable, and a conclusion. The inquiry table always displays the worksheet state corresponding to the current state of the video: Each time one of the learners starts to take notes about their current experiment, all the information that is written down at this point is displayed at once so that the pre-service teachers can immediately process this information. This information enables the pre-service teachers to keep track of the experiments the students have already conducted.

3. The bottom-right area ("note pad") comprises a text box for notes participants can write down while watching the video, just as teachers could take notes during their lessons. In some versions of the simulation environment the note pad contains some text that structures the pre-service teachers' notes. The notes are saved and displayed again later when participants write their final diagnosis.
4. The bottom-left area ("navigation area") displays questions ("video links") that serve as links to short video segments that can be inserted at certain points of the main video and that contain a voice-over of a teacher asking the respective question to the learners in the video along with their responses.

Video Material The videos show a classroom situation focused on two students. Several scripted videos were produced that show these students performing two inquiry tasks. The tasks are based on the two already described scientific experiments. The physics experiment has to do with lenses and the biology experiment has to do with the growth of plants. Both experiments have exactly the same structure. In both cases, the learners in the video have to find out whether and how the dependent variables—plant growth and optimal distance between lens and illustration screen, respectively—are influenced by four independent variables. In physics, the four independent variables are (1) the curvature of the lens, (2) the size of the lens, (3) the distance between the object and the lens, and (4) a so-called polarizing filter. In biology, the four variables are (1) the amount of water, (2) salt, (3) a fertilizer stick, and (4) an unspecified white powder. The videos are the pre-service teachers' main source of information, supplemented only by the inquiry table that documents the learners' experiments.

Developing Video Scripts At the beginning of creating the simulations, we came up with and wrote down several fictional student profiles containing appropriate values for all relevant scientific reasoning subskills, with the objective of creating realistic, average students. We then wrote corresponding scripts matching these profiles. Those scripts were later handed to the student actors to prepare for their roles and learn their dialogues.

Interaction By default, typical media player control elements (e.g., play, pause, stop, forward, backward, replay, and time bar functionalities as well as a time display) are disabled for the video area. Thus, the simulation platform mimics the situation in classroom instruction, during which there is also no opportunity to interrupt or revisit parts of the flow of events. To be sure, video interactivity and reflection phases may be helpful design features of video simulations, which can also be investigated in this simulation environment.

The video links in the navigation area constitute the essential feature of the environment that renders it a simulation, because they enable the participants to "interact with the students" in the videos (see Fig. 7.2). During the planning and documentation phases of each experiment in the video, groups of video links with questions that might be appropriate at this point are displayed in the navigation area.

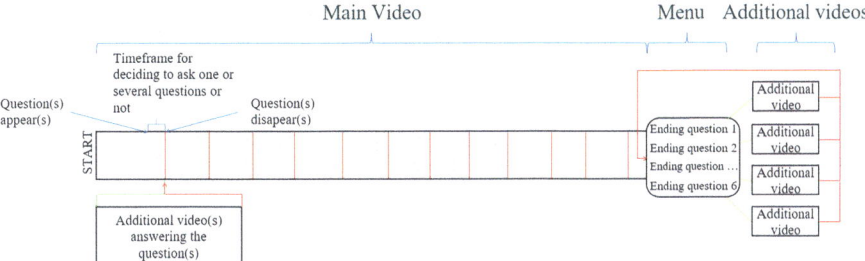

Fig. 7.2 Flowchart for the simulations

When the learners run the experiment or move on to the next experiment, the group of video links disappears and is eventually replaced by a new group of video links.

If a participant decides to ask a certain question (for example: "What do you want to find out now?"), he or she may click on the corresponding link. The video segment containing the teacher question and learner response is then inserted at the next appropriate point in the main video following the selection of the corresponding question. Until this point, participants have the possibility to withdraw their selection by clicking on the video link for a second time. They may also select more than one video link. If the participant has selected several video links, the corresponding video segments are played in a prespecified sequence. After choosing a question and watching the additional video segment, the main video continues. Only the remaining video links are displayed; hence, no video segment can be viewed twice.

After the main video has ended, a group of video links is displayed that comprises questions which do not refer to individual experiments, but rather to the sequence of experiments as a whole (see Fig. 7.2). One example of these ending questions is: "Is there one or even more than one experiment that wasn't completely necessary and therefore could have been left out?" When the participant selects one of these video links, the video segment with the corresponding question is played immediately. After the video segment has ended, again only the remaining video links are displayed, and the next question can be selected.

The participants have only limited time for questions during each simulation. It is therefore impossible to view all additional video segments. Hence, participants have to choose the most relevant and important ones. These interactions should always serve the purpose of gaining additional relevant information about the learner's scientific reasoning skills that cannot be obtained from the main video. In some cases, it also makes sense to postpone the selection of a specific question because the corresponding information may occur in the main video at some later point, and only ask the question at a later occasion if it turns out that the main video does not contain the information. To help the participants keep track of the available time, both the time remaining for additional questions and the length of the video segments corresponding to the video links are displayed in the navigation area.

7.1.5 Measuring Pre-Service Teachers' Diagnostic Activities and the Quality of Their Diagnoses of Students' Scientific Reasoning Skills

The participants' performance in the simulation is later evaluated using accuracy and efficiency measures. Accuracy is a measure for the quality of the participants' performance in the simulations in terms of choosing the "right" questions. Therefore, we consider the "right" questions to be those that are promising in the sense of the expectation to provide useful information for the diagnosing process. Since we additionally need some unimportant questions as distractors, there are also some questions that are either completely irrelevant or focused on information that can easily be acquired just by watching the main video. On the other hand, efficiency is a measure of accuracy in proportion to time. This is important because participants are encouraged to use their time for questions wisely.

In addition to the performance evaluation in the simulations, we also evaluate the participants' written diagnoses using only a measure of accuracy. Both the individual diagnoses and—in the collaborative test condition—the additional collaborative diagnoses are rated by comparing them to a sample solution. This sample solution is based on the student profiles used to create the scripts, which include the envisaged values for all relevant scientific reasoning subskills. The level of congruence between the sample solution and the individual diagnosis is considered as an accuracy measure.

7.1.6 Research on (Support for) Pre-Service Teachers' Diagnosis of Students' Scientific Reasoning Skills in Video-Based Simulations

The simulation environment and the video simulations described in this contribution provide a basis for investigating several important research questions concerning pre-service teachers' diagnosis of students' scientific reasoning skills. In our research, we focus on two main areas: The role of different types and content-related facets of professional knowledge for (pre-service) teachers' diagnostic activities and the quality of diagnoses of students' scientific reasoning skills on the one hand, and on kinds of scaffolding that foster the development of pre-service teachers' individual and collaborative diagnostic competences concerning students' scientific reasoning skills in video-based simulations on the other. Putting our research interests in context, we will focus on Research Questions 2 and 4, as mentioned in both the introduction by Fischer et al. (2022) and the concluding chapter by Opitz et al. (2022). In particular, we investigate

1. how conceptual content knowledge, scientific reasoning skills, and conceptual pedagogical content knowledge about scientific reasoning and its diagnosis among pre-service teachers in physics and biology are related to their diagnostic activities and the quality of their diagnoses,
2. how the collaborative vs. individual development of a diagnosis influences diagnostic activities and the quality of the diagnosis, as well as what role the distribution of information (shared vs. separate experiences of learners' inquiry activities during lessons) plays in this respect, and,
3. to what extent a collaboration script for joint diagnosis can enhance diagnostic activities and the quality of the diagnosis as well as the development of individual and collaborative diagnostic competences.

Thus, in the long run, the present research may contribute to the improvement of teacher education at universities.

Acknowledgments The research presented in this chapter was funded by a grant from the Deutsche Forschungsgemeinschaft (DFG-FOR 2385) to Christof Wecker, Birgit Neuhaus, and Raimund Girwidz (WE 5426/2-1).

References

Baumert, J., & Kunter, M. (2006). Stichwort: Professionelle Kompetenz von Lehrkräften. *Zeitschrift für Erziehungswissenschaft, 9*, 469–520. https://doi.org/10.1007/s11618-006-0165-2

Chen, Z., & Klahr, D. (1999). All other things being equal: Acquisition and transfer of the control of variables strategy. *Child Development, 70*, 1098–1120. https://doi.org/10.1111/1467-8624.00081

Chernikova, O., Heitzmann, N., Opitz, A., Seidel, T., & Fischer, F. (2022). A theoretical framework for fostering diagnostic competences with simulations. In F. Fischer & A. Opitz (Eds.), *Learning to diagnose with simulations—Examples from teacher education and medical education*. Springer.

de Jong, T. (2006). Computer simulations. Technological advances in inquiry learning. *Science, 312*, 532–533. https://doi.org/10.1126/science.1127750

de Jong, T., & van Joolingen, W. R. (1998). Scientific discovery learning with computer simulations of conceptual domains. *Review of Educational Research, 68*, 179–201. https://doi.org/10.2307/1170753

de Wit, F. R. C., & Greer, L. L. (2008). The black-box deciphered: A meta-analysis of team diversity, conflict, and team performance. In *Academy of management proceedings* (Vol. 1, pp. 1–6). Academy of Management.

Fischer, F., Kollar, I., Ufer, S., Sodian, B., Hussmann, H., Pekrun, R., et al. (2014). Scientific reasoning and argumentation: Advancing an interdisciplinary research agenda in education. *Frontline Learning Research, 2*(3), 28–45.

Fischer, F., Chernikova, O., & Opitz, A. (2022). Learning to diagnose with simulations: Introduction. In F. Fischer & A. Opitz (Eds.), *Learning to diagnose with simulations—examples from teacher education and medical education*. Springer.

Förtsch, C., Sommerhoff, D., Fischer, F., Fischer, M., Girwidz, R., Obersteiner, A., et al. (2018). Systematizing professional knowledge of medical doctors and teachers: Development of an interdisciplinary framework in the context of diagnostic competences. *Educational Sciences, 8*, 207. https://doi.org/10.3390/educsci8040207

Hautz, W. E., Kämmer, J. E., Schauber, S. K., Spies, C. D., & Gaissmaier, W. (2015). Diagnostic performance by medical students working individually or in teams. *JAMA, 313,* 303–304. https://doi.org/10.1001/jama.2014.15770

Heitzmann, N., Seidel, T., Opitz, A., Hetmanek, A., Wecker, C., Fischer, M., et al. (2019). Facilitating diagnostic competences in simulations in higher education. *Frontline Learning Research, 7*(4), 1–24. https://doi.org/10.14786/flr.v7i4.384

Helmke, A. (2010). *Unterrichtsqualität und Lehrerprofessionalität: Diagnose, Evaluation und Verbesserung des Unterrichts* (3rd ed.). Klett Kallmeyer.

Hetmanek, A., Engelman, K., Opitz, A., & Fischer, F. (2018). Beyond intelligence and domain knowledge: Scientific reasoning and argumentation as a set of cross-domain skills. In F. Fischer, C. A. Chinn, K. F. Engelmann, & J. Osborne (Eds.), *Scientific reasoning and argumentation: The roles of domain-specific and domain-general knowledge* (pp. 203–226). Routledge.

Hilbert, T. S., Nückles, M., Renkl, A., Minarik, C., Reich, A., & Ruhe, K. (2008). Concept Mapping zum Lernen aus Texten. *Zeitschrift für Pädagogische Psychologie, 22,* 119–125. https://doi.org/10.1024/1010-0652.22.2.119

Klahr, D., & Dunbar, K. (1988). Dual space search during scientific reasoning. *Cognitive Science, 12,* 1–48.

Koeppen, K., Hartig, J., Klieme, E., & Leutner, D. (2008). Current issues in competence modeling and assessment. *Zeitschrift für Psychologie/Journal of Psychology, 216,* 61–73. https://doi.org/10.1027/0044-3409.216.2.61

Kuhn, D., Schauble, L., & Garcia-Mila, M. (1992). Cross-domain development of scientific reasoning. *Cognition and Instruction, 9,* 285–327. https://doi.org/10.1207/s1532690xci0904_1

Lazonder, A. W., Wilhelm, P., & Hagemans, M. G. (2008). The influence of domain knowledge on strategy use during simulation-based inquiry learning. *Learning and Instruction, 18,* 580–592. https://doi.org/10.1016/j.learninstruc.2007.12.001

Opitz, A., Fischer, M., Seidel, T., & Fischer, F. (2022). Conclusions and outlook: Toward more systematic research on the use of simulations in higher education. In F. Fischer & A. Opitz (Eds.), *Learning to diagnose with simulations—Examples from teacher education and medical education.* Springer.

Osborne, J. (2018). Styles of scientific reasoning: What can we learn from looking at the product, not the process, of scientific reasoning? In F. Fischer, C. A. Chinn, K. F. Engelmann, & J. Osborne (Eds.), *Scientific reasoning and argumentation: The roles of domain-specific and domain-general knowledge* (pp. 162–186). Routledge.

Peeraer, G., Scherpbier, A. J., Remmen, R., de Winder, B. Y., Hendrickx, K., van Petegem, P., et al. (2007). Clinical skills training in a skills lab compared with skills training in internships: Comparison of skills development curricula. *Education and Health, 20*(3), 125.

Radkowitsch, A., Sailer, M., Fischer, M. R., Schmidmaier, R., & Fischer, F. (2022). Diagnosing collaboratively: A theoretical model and a simulation-based learning environment. In F. Fischer & A. Opitz (Eds.), *Learning to diagnose with simulations—Examples from teacher education and medical education.* Springer.

Renkl, A., Hilbert, T., & Schworm, S. (2009). Example-based learning in heuristic domains: A cognitive load theory account. *Educational Psychology Review, 21,* 67–78. https://doi.org/10.1007/s10648-008-9093-4

Schrader, F.-W. (2009). Anmerkungen zum Themenschwerpunkt Diagnostische Kompetenz von Lehrkräften. *Zeitschrift für Pädagogische Psychologie, 23,* 237–245. https://doi.org/10.1024/1010-0652.23.34.237

Schunn, C. D., & Anderson, J. R. (1999). The generality/specificity of expertise in scientific reasoning. *Cognitive Science, 23,* 337–370. https://doi.org/10.1207/s15516709cog2303_3

Schwichow, M., Christoph, S., Boone, W. J., & Härtig, H. (2016). The impact of sub-skills and item content on students' skills with regard to the control-of-variables strategy. *International Journal of Science Education, 38,* 216–237. https://doi.org/10.1080/09500693.2015.1137651

Südkamp, A., Kaiser, J., & Möller, J. (2012). Accuracy of teachers' judgments of students' academic achievement: A meta-analysis. *Journal of Educational Psychology, 104*, 743–762. https://doi.org/10.1037/a0027627

Tricot, A., & Sweller, J. (2014). Domain-specific knowledge and why teaching generic skills does not work. *Educational Psychology Review, 26*, 265–283. https://doi.org/10.1007/s10648-013-9243-1

Tschirgi, J. E. (1980). Sensible reasoning: A hypothesis about hypotheses. *Child Development, 51*(1), 1–10.

VanLehn, K. (1996). Cognitive skill acquisition. *Annual Review of Psychology, 47*, 513–539. https://doi.org/10.1146/annurev.psych.47.1.513

Wecker, C., Hetmanek, A., & Fischer, F. (2016). Zwei Fliegen mit einer Klappe? Fachwissen und fächerübergreifende Kompetenzen gemeinsam fördern. *Unterrichtswissenschaft, 44*(3), 226–238.

Zimmerman, C. (2007). The development of scientific thinking skills in elementary and middle school. *Developmental Review, 27*, 172–223. https://doi.org/10.1016/j.dr.2006.12.001

Open Access This chapter is licensed under the terms of the Creative Commons Attribution 4.0 International License (http://creativecommons.org/licenses/by/4.0/), which permits use, sharing, adaptation, distribution and reproduction in any medium or format, as long as you give appropriate credit to the original author(s) and the source, provide a link to the Creative Commons license and indicate if changes were made.

The images or other third party material in this chapter are included in the chapter's Creative Commons license, unless indicated otherwise in a credit line to the material. If material is not included in the chapter's Creative Commons license and your intended use is not permitted by statutory regulation or exceeds the permitted use, you will need to obtain permission directly from the copyright holder.

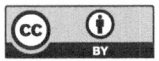

Chapter 8
Learning to Diagnose Students' Behavioral, Developmental, and Learning Disorders in a Simulation-Based Learning Environment for Pre-Service Teachers

Elisabeth Bauer, Michael Sailer, Jan Kiesewetter, Claudia Schulz, Iryna Gurevych, Martin R. Fischer, and Frank Fischer

This chapter's simulation at a glance

Domain	Teacher education
Topic	Students' behavioral, developmental, and learning disorders
Learner's task	Take on the role of a teacher and gather information about a problematic student to identify if the student may have a clinically relevant disorder and if so, which one it could be
Target group	Pre-service teachers for all school tracks in various stages of teacher education
Diagnostic mode	Individual diagnosing
Sources of information	Documents (students' school assignments, report cards, etc.); reports of the student's in-class and out-of-class behavior; protocols of conversations with other teachers, the student and parents
Special features	Use of natural language processing to provide automatic adaptive feedback based on the learners' written explanations of their diagnostic conclusion and processing of the case

---

E. Bauer (✉) · M. Sailer · F. Fischer
Chair of Education and Educational Psychology, Department of Psychology, LMU Munich, Munich, Germany
e-mail: Elisabeth.Bauer@psy.lmu.de

J. Kiesewetter · M. R. Fischer
Institute for Medical Education, University Hospital, LMU Munich, Munich, Germany

C. Schulz · I. Gurevych
Ubiquitous Knowledge Processing (UKP) Lab, Department of Computer Science, Technical University Darmstadt, Darmstadt, Germany

© The Authors(s) 2022
F. Fischer, A. Opitz (eds.), *Learning to Diagnose with Simulations*,
https://doi.org/10.1007/978-3-030-89147-3_8

8.1 Competence Goals in Higher Education

Contemporary curricula in higher education emphasize the need to facilitate students' competence development. This trend is supported by practitioners and politicians, arguing that work in the digital age requires not merely conceptual knowledge but also the ability to apply it to complex tasks in ill-defined situations (Ananiadou & Claro, 2009). The emphasis on diagnostic competence development in medical and teacher education is one of many examples related to this trend. In accordance with Fischer et al. (2022), we define the action of diagnosing as the goal-oriented collection and interpretation of case-specific or problem-specific information to reduce uncertainty in order to make medical or educational decisions. Thus, diagnostic competences are indicated by the accuracy of the diagnosis, application of professional knowledge (see Förtsch et al., 2018), and performance of appropriate epistemic-diagnostic activities (see Fischer et al., 2014).

Since learning competences is highly complex, support structures are required that guide learners in their learning process (Chernikova et al., 2022; Van Merriënboer et al., 2002). One such support structure is feedback, which has been shown to be one of the main predictors of learning outcomes (Hattie & Timperley, 2007). Individual feedback requires high time investments by higher education instructors, which is why it is often neglected (Nicol, 2010). This is one example of how changing professional requirements affect learning objectives, which in turn affect higher education practices and requirements.

Simultaneously, digitalization has brought about technical innovations that can help to facilitate the adaptation of higher education practices. In recent decades, computer-supported and web-based learning has enabled the widespread usage of a range of instructional methods and measures for learning support. Among these is simulation-based learning (Baek, 2009; Gegenfurtner et al., 2014), which has been shown to be an effective approach for competence development (Berman et al., 2016). There are also attempts to automate learner support in digital learning environments, such as using artificial intelligence for intelligent tutoring systems (Diziol et al., 2010; Naser, 2012). Such intelligent systems are able to adapt automatically to learners' competence level and learning progress by automatically analyzing log data. Novel approaches also automate the analysis of written answers using natural language processing (NLP) methods. These systems are utilized, for example, to analyze lexical, syntactical, rhetorical, and other features of learners' essays to provide feedback on the essays' quality in terms of writing strategy (McNamara et al., 2013). A more detailed automated analysis of writing strategy in combination with the content of written answers was previously unrealizable due to limitations of natural language processing methods (Diziol et al., 2010).

FAMULUS makes progress on this technical challenge with the most recent natural language processing methodology, namely artificial neural networks, to provide automatic adaptive feedback on learners' written text answers while they are engaged in simulation-based learning, in order to foster their diagnostic competences. The feedback is conceptualized to consider both the strategy and content applied in the text answers. This combination better approximates more advanced levels of feedback. Moreover, FAMULUS is an interdisciplinary project involving the disciplines of teacher and medical education. The current chapter gives an overview of the project's background, goals, learning environment, schedule and open questions referring to the teacher education subproject.

8.2 Teachers' Diagnosing of Their Students' Psychological Problems

As previous chapters have already outlined (see Chernikova et al., 2022; Codreanu et al., 2022), diagnostic competences are a core learning objective in teacher education. Teachers have to diagnose students' performance (Schrader, 2011) and individual prerequisites, such as competence level and motivation (Spinath, 2005). These individual prerequisites also include students' behavioral, developmental, and learning disorders. Such disorders affect around 5% of students (Hölling et al., 2014). Behavioral disorders like ADHD and developmental disorders like specific learning disorders become observable in elementary school or early secondary school at the latest and are therefore relevant for teachers in all types of schools. Often, the symptomatology further evolves as students face increasing performance-related and social challenges in school (Schulte-Körne, 2016). This is why teachers are confronted with students' behavioral, developmental, and learning disorders in their classrooms. They are oftentimes the first professionals who have the opportunity to identify an existing problem and initiate further action (Reinke et al., 2011). Therefore, diagnosing students' psychological problems is not only a relevant aspect of teachers' everyday practice but part of their professional responsibility. When confronted with a problem, teachers need to apply epistemic activities, like generating hypotheses, generating and evaluating evidence for and against these hypotheses, and drawing diagnostic conclusions (see Fischer et al., 2014). In this regard, diagnosing can be decomposed into the application of a diagnostic strategy (see Fischer et al., 2014) and relevant concept knowledge (see Coderre et al., 2003; see Förtsch et al., 2018). One example would be the evaluation of the evidence for "inattention" and "hyperactivity" to draw a conclusion regarding the hypothesis "ADHD". Teachers should be able to identify psychological problems among students and apply a diagnostic strategy and relevant concepts accordingly. Moreover, they need to be able to communicate their diagnoses professionally (see Lawson & Daniel, 2011) e.g., to a school psychologist. This requires combining arguments for and (if applicable) against differential diagnoses to construct a diagnostic argument.

Despite its relevance, students' psychological problems are rarely part of teachers' initial professional education. It has been found that teachers rate their general knowledge about psychological disorders as mediocre at best (Reinke et al.,

2011; Rothì et al., 2008). Consequently, diagnosing students' psychological problems seems to be a particular challenge for teachers (Eklund et al., 2009; Papandrea & Winefield, 2011; Rothì et al., 2008; Trudgen & Lawn, 2011). Aside from students' families, teachers usually possess the broadest information about individual students. Observations in and outside the classroom, documents like assignments and exams, conversations with other teachers, the students themselves, parents or other students can provide meaningful insights. Moreover, teachers can observe their students over the course of at least one school year and therefore gain a developmental perspective on each student. In particular, externalizing disorders like ADHD that manifest considerably in a student's behavior allow teachers to apply a wide range of observational methods and resources. Other disorders that can be identified by teachers are developmental disorders of scholastic skills like dyslexia, since they have a strong impact on a student's performance.

Generally, the literature on teachers' diagnosing of students' psychological problems is sparse. One reason for that might be that the topic is located at the intersection of two professional disciplines, namely teaching and clinical psychology. These two disciplines as well as adjacent professional disciplines offer valuable insights into teachers' diagnosing and how to design a suitable learning environment for pre-service teachers. The following section further elaborates on the interdisciplinary relations concerning teachers' diagnosing of students' psychological problems.

8.3 Interdisciplinary Setting

The central discipline with respect to designing a simulation and learning environment that aims to improve teachers' diagnostic competences is of course teacher education. It is important to understand that diagnosing students' psychological problems is only one among many demands teachers are asked to fulfill in their everyday practice. Therefore, realistic learning objectives must first be determined. It seems reasonable to suggest that teachers should be able to identify students' psychological problems in terms of distinguishing between clinically relevant and nonrelevant behavior, reflect on potential hypotheses and generate, evaluate, and integrate evidence obtainable in the everyday school setting. Therefore, the learning goal is the capability to draw substantiated conclusions and formulate argumentation texts to communicate these conclusions to other teachers and psychological professionals.

The distinction between clinically relevant and nonrelevant behavior and the classification of symptoms in terms of disorders are closely related to the discipline of clinical psychology. These concepts build on diagnostic categories defined by the medical domain and documented in diagnostic manuals such as the ICD-10 (Dilling et al., 2015), which serves as the diagnostic reference standard in Germany. To achieve the aforementioned learning goal, pre-service teacher education needs to provide basic conceptual knowledge on diagnostic classifications and related symptomatology that are particularly relevant for the age group served by a given school type. Moreover, some general strategic knowledge on how to approach diagnosing, generate evidence, and differentiate between different diagnoses with similar manifestations is necessary.

To design an effective learning environment that targets teachers' diagnostic competences, research on diagnostic processes and actions should be taken into account. Such research can primarily be found in the discipline of medical education. A central insight in this field is that learning how to apply conceptual diagnostic knowledge and diagnostic strategy based on case information requires repeated practice (Schmidt & Rikers, 2007). In medical education, this practice is commonly provided by confronting learners with virtual patients (Berman et al., 2016). Educators present virtual patients in different presentation formats. One such format is the serial cue format, which presents case information separated by units. Typically, the case information is presented as the results of various medical tests, which can be accessed in a sequential fashion.

8.4 Simulation Description

FAMULUS designs and tests a learning environment involving document-based simulation to foster diagnostic competences. The learning environment is implemented using the learning management system CASUS (Simonsohn & Fischer, 2004). Building on the idea of virtual patients, the learning environment presents six cases of students showing problems that are potentially related to a behavioral, developmental or learning disorder. The cases were developed with the involvement of experts in school psychology and educational sciences. Blueprints were created before the case information was divided up and assigned to informational sources like "classroom observation" or "meeting with parents". Based on the blueprints, different types of learning materials were developed, e.g., written records of conversations or observations and visuals of documents, such as report cards and school assignments. Following this procedure, six cases in the serial cue format were designed and implemented in the simulation-based learning environment. Another expert from psychotherapy validated the cases in terms of symptomatic authenticity and representativeness.

During the learning phase, learners first watch a 20-min video presenting basic knowledge about diagnosing and behavioral, developmental, and learning disorders among students. This video was included to meet learners' prerequisites (see Chernikova et al., 2022) by addressing their limited prior professional knowledge base. Next, learners are asked to adopt the perspective of a teacher and diagnose the six learning cases. While interacting with the learning environment, they need to apply four epistemic activities in particular (Chernikova et al., 2022; Fischer et al., 2014): generating hypotheses, generating evidence, evaluating evidence and drawing conclusions. For each case, they receive brief initial problem information. On this basis, the learners need to generate up to three initial hypotheses. They then can access the complete case information, which is presented in serial cue format with the following informational sources: the teacher's classroom observations, schoolyard observations, school assignments and report cards as well as conversations with other fictional teachers, the student him- or herself and the student's parents. The learners do not have to examine all informational sources but make selections and stop the information search at any time. Thus, the learning environment simulates the activities of evidence generation and evaluation. As a final task for each case, learners have to draw a diagnostic conclusion. Moreover, they are asked to communicate their diagnostic actions and write a substantiated argumentation text for their conclusion in a free-text format.

8.5 Feedback Description

As part of the learning environment, an automatic adaptive feedback tool was designed as a learner support (see Chernikova et al., 2022). It specifically addresses the gap between a learner's answer and the sample solution for each learning case and provides hints on how to better apply relevant conceptual and strategic knowledge. Providing such process-related explanations which point the learners to individual options for improvement has been shown to be more effective for learning competences than simpler feedback like presenting the correct response—e.g., an expert solution (Hattie & Timperley, 2007).

Learners receive automatic adaptive feedback on their diagnostic argumentation texts. The feedback is given on two levels: the application of a diagnostic strategy and the application of case-specific concepts. The general diagnostic strategy refers to the epistemic activities of generating hypotheses, generating evidence, evaluating evidence and drawing conclusions (Fischer et al., 2014). The case-specific concepts concern differential hypotheses in the clinical spectrum (e.g., ADHD) as well as hypotheses in the nonclinical spectrum (e.g., family problems), and particular evidence (e.g., inattention, hyperactivity and impulsivity). To provide in-time automatic adaptive feedback, the learners' argumentation texts are automatically analyzed by an NLP algorithm, more specifically an artificial neural network (Schulz et al., 2019). The algorithm automatically identifies the presence or absence of the four epistemic activities and several case-specific concepts. It does so by calculating the likelihood of expressions' affiliation to previously trained categories. This enables the algorithm to automatically analyze new texts and recognize unknown expressions, which, however, need to be similar to what the algorithm learned earlier. This automatic analysis, in turn, activates a range of predefined feedback components. These components combine to form a real-time automatic adaptive feedback response for each learner's argumentation text for each learning case.

If, for example, a learner did not draw a diagnostic conclusion in their argumentation text, he or she receives the feedback that this component is essential but missing in their submitted argumentation text. The learner is also prompted to include a substantiated conclusion in their next argumentation text. One example for feedback on the conceptual level would be the confirmation of correctly considered diagnoses and the correction of incorrectly considered diagnoses as well as feedback on specific evidence used to justify the arguments.

The overall quality of the adaptive feedback critically depends on how accurately the NLP algorithm detects epistemic activities and case-specific concepts. The following section further illustrates the associated tasks and challenges for the project, referring to the example of automatically analyzing epistemic activities.

8.6 Training of an NLP Algorithm

Previous studies have already attempted to train NLP algorithms for the automatic identification of epistemic activities (Daxenberger et al., 2018). These algorithms were trained based on the coding of think-aloud protocols of pre-service teachers diagnosing everyday classroom problems (Csanadi et al., 2016) and social workers diagnosing client problems (Ghanem et al., 2018). These studies applied the method of conditional random fields (CRFs; Okazaki, 2007). CRFs consider the correlations between adjacent codes to identify the best chain of codes for each sentence (Ma & Hovy, 2016). However, the accuracy of the algorithms in identifying epistemic activities was rather weak.

The FAMULUS algorithm is trained based on argumentation text data collected in the context of a previous study. This previous study had 118 pre-service teachers learn with a preliminary version of the FAMULUS simulation-based learning environment involving the six current learning cases and two additional cases from the same symptomatic spectrum. The resulting data set of 944 argumentation texts was manually coded by four coders concerning the four epistemic activities of generating hypotheses, generating evidence, evaluating evidence and drawing conclusions. The intercoder reliability was calculated based on 150 fourfold-coded texts, resulting in sufficient agreement.

Based on a data set of 440 argumentation texts, a first neural network model was fitted. The CRF method was combined with the more recent method of bidirectional long short-term memory (BILSTM; Reimers & Gurevych, 2017). The BILSTM method considers the overall context of codes within the text by looking at bidirectional long-term dependencies (Ma & Hovy, 2016). Schulz et al. (2019) provide further details about the methodology and model fitting process.

The performance of the algorithm was tested on 110 additional argumentation texts, showing a satisfactory model fit. The algorithm's coding performance was also compared to the human intercoder reliability and achieved more than 70% of the human coding performance. Moreover, the FAMULUS algorithm achieved almost twice the performance reported by previous studies attempting to train algorithms for the automatic identification of epistemic activities (Daxenberger et al., 2018).

In the future, the training data set for the algorithm will be extended to the full data set of 944 argumentation texts. The algorithm will also be extended to automatically code the dimension of case-specific concepts. The extended and improved algorithm will then serve as a basis for the automatic adaptive feedback component.

8.7 Outlook

In an upcoming laboratory study, the automatic adaptive feedback will be compared with a nonadaptive feedback option regarding the effect on learning diagnostic competences. In doing so, we will contribute to Questions 2 (learner support) and 4 (adaptation) of the overarching research questions mentioned in the introduction by Fischer et al. (2022). The proposed sample for the study consists of 180 pre-service teachers. They will access the learning environment, diagnose the six simulated learning cases and write an argumentation text for every case. Participants in the experimental condition will receive adaptive feedback in line with their argumentation texts, while participants in the control group will receive static feedback consisting of a comprehensive expert solution. The effects of both types of feedback will be analyzed regarding several outcomes: (1) diagnostic accuracy in the learning cases and (2) knowledge gain from pre- to post-test. It is expected that the automatic adaptive feedback will exceed the nonadaptive expert solution in terms of participants' performance and learning gains.

This experimental study will be replicated in a second FAMULUS sub-project that develops a highly similar learning environment and adaptive feedback component to foster diagnostic competences in medical education. In the medical learning environment, learners will have to diagnose six patients with symptoms of fever or back pain. An interdisciplinary comparison of the sub-projects from teacher and medical education regarding learners' interactions with the learning environment and the structure of their diagnostic argumentations might reveal interesting results as well. One example would be to explore sequences of epistemic activities in diagnostic argumentation (see Csanadi et al., 2018). The sequence of epistemic activities seems to differ substantially across pre-service teachers. A comparison with medical students might indicate interdisciplinary similarities or differences in the variability and predominant patterns of sequences. Moreover, changes in variability and sequences across the learning cases will be examined.

Another area of exploration is how to further improve the NLP algorithm's coding accuracy. The accuracy generally depends on several determinants, such as the consistency and quality of the text material, the amount of training data, the consistency and quality of the training data, and consistency of the coding in the training data. One solution approach within the FAMULUS project is an attempt to improve the consistency and quality of the text material that has to be coded. The previously collected text material currently being used as training data will be analyzed in terms of the potential need to further clarify the task instructions. Improving the instructions (if necessary) might in turn improve the consistency and quality of the argumentation texts collected in the upcoming study and hence future additional NLP training data. Adding argumentation texts from the upcoming study to the training data will also increase the overall amount of training data. These steps might further increase the algorithm's accuracy and thus also the quality and effectiveness of the automatic adaptive feedback.

Lastly, it will be interesting to examine how the FAMULUS learning environment can be integrated into actual higher education classes. This transfer will be investigated in a field study. This simulation-based learning opportunity will be offered in regular teacher education classes at three different universities. The implementation will be evaluated and the results of the laboratory studies will be validated.

8.8 Conclusion

Simulation-based learning is a feasible approach to implement effective learning environments in higher education for competences, such as diagnostic competences. However, learning competences requires specific and intensive learner support. Implementing high-quality learner support that can be feasibly applied on a large scale is a major challenge. Automation using artificial intelligence seems to be a promising way to approach some parts of these challenges. FAMULUS illustrates and evaluates natural language processing measures to automate process-related feedback on diagnostic argumentation text answers. Some initial applications of the natural language processing algorithms presented in this chapter indicate that the automated text analyses might be sufficiently accurate to support learners with adaptive process-related feedback during their learning. This appears to be particularly important in interdisciplinary and ill-defined fields of application like teachers' diagnosing of students' behavioral, developmental, and learning disorders, where corresponding learning opportunities are largely lacking or neglect competence-oriented learning.

Acknowledgments This research was supported by a grant from the German Federal Ministry of Research and Education (Grant No.: 16DHL1039).

References

Ananiadou, K., & Claro, M. (2009). *21st century skills and competences for new millennium learners in OECD countries*. OECD.
Baek, Y. (2009). Digital simulation in teaching and learning. In *Digital simulations for improving education: Learning through artificial teaching environments* (pp. 25–51). IGI Global.
Berman, N. B., Durning, S. J., Fischer, M. R., Huwendiek, S., & Triola, M. M. (2016). The role for virtual patients in the future of medical education. *Academic Medicine, 91*(9), 1217–1222.
Chernikova, O., Heitzmann, N., Opitz, A., & Fischer, F. (2022). A theoretical framework for fostering diagnostic competences with simulations. In F. Fischer & A. Opitz (Eds.), *Learning to diagnose with simulations—Examples from teacher education and medical education*. Springer.
Coderre, S., Mandin, H., Harasym, P. H., & Fick, G. H. (2003). Diagnostic reasoning strategies and diagnostic success. *Medical Education, 37*(8), 695–703.
Codreanu, E., Huber, S., Reinhold, S., Sommerhoff, D., Neuhaus, B., Schmidmaier, R., & Seidel, T. (2022). Diagnosing mathematical argumentation skills: A video-based simulation for pre-service teachers. In F. Fischer & A. Opitz (Eds.), *Learning to diagnose with simulations—examples from teacher education and medical education*. Springer.

Csanadi, A., Kollar, I., & Fischer, F. (2016). *Scientific reasoning and problem-solving in a practical domain: Are two heads better than one?* International Society of the Learning Sciences.

Csanadi, A., Eagan, B., Kollar, I., Shaffer, D. W., & Fischer, F. (2018). When coding-and-counting is not enough: Using epistemic network analysis (ENA) to analyze verbal data in CSCL research. *International Journal of Computer-Supported Collaborative Learning, 13*(4), 419–438.

Daxenberger, J., Csanadi, A., Ghanem, C., Kollar, I., & Gurevych, I. (2018). Domain-specific aspects of scientific reasoning and argumentation: Insights from automatic coding. In *Scientific reasoning and argumentation* (pp. 44–65). Routledge.

Dilling, H., Mombour, W., & Schmidt, M. H. (2015). Internationale Klassifikation psychischer Störungen. In *ICD-10 Kapitel V (F). Klinisch-diagnostische Leitlinien* (10th ed.). Hogrefe.

Diziol, D., Walker, E., Rummel, N., & Koedinger, K. R. (2010). Using intelligent tutor technology to implement adaptive support for student collaboration. *Educational Psychology Review, 22*(1), 89–102.

Eklund, K., Renshaw, T. L., Dowdy, E., Jimerson, S. R., Hart, S. R., Jones, C. N., & Earhart, J. (2009). Early identification of behavioral and emotional problems in youth: Universal screening versus teacher-referral identification. *The California School Psychologist, 14*, 89–95.

Fischer, F., Kollar, I., Ufer, S., Sodian, B., Hussmann, H., Pekrun, R., Fischer, M., et al. (2014). Scientific reasoning and argumentation: Advancing an interdisciplinary research agenda in education. *Frontline Learning Research, 2*(3), 28–45.

Fischer, F., Chernikova, O., & Opitz, A. (2022). Learning to diagnose with simulations: Introduction. In F. Fischer & A. Opitz (Eds.), *Learning to diagnose with simulations—examples from teacher education and medical education*. Springer.

Förtsch, C., Sommerhoff, D., Fischer, F., Fischer, M., Girwidz, R., Obersteiner, A., Schmidmaier, R., et al. (2018). Systematizing professional knowledge of medical doctors and teachers: Development of an interdisciplinary framework in the context of diagnostic competences. *Educational Sciences, 8*(4), 207.

Gegenfurtner, A., Quesada-Pallarès, C., & Knogler, M. (2014). Digital simulation-based training: A meta-analysis. *British Journal of Educational Technology, 45*(6), 1097–1114.

Ghanem, C., Kollar, I., Fischer, F., Lawson, T. R., & Pankofer, S. (2018). How do social work novices and experts solve professional problems? A micro-analysis of epistemic activities and the use of evidence. *European Journal of Social Work, 21*(1), 3–19.

Hattie, J., & Timperley, H. (2007). The power of feedback. *Review of Educational Research, 77*(1), 81–112.

Hölling, H., Schlack, R., Petermann, F., Ravens-Sieberer, U., Mauz, E., & Group, K. S. (2014). Psychische Auffälligkeiten und psychosoziale Beeinträchtigungen bei Kindern und Jugendlichen im Alter von 3 bis 17 Jahren in Deutschland–Prävalenz und zeitliche Trends zu 2 Erhebungszeitpunkten (2003–2006 und 2009–2012) [Psychological and psychosocial problems of German children and adolescents from age of 3 to 17—Prevalences and temporal trends of 2 measurement points (2003–2006 und 2009–2012)]. *Bundesgesundheitsblatt - Gesundheitsforschung - Gesundheitsschutz, 57*(7), 807–819.

Lawson, A. E., & Daniel, E. S. (2011). Inferences of clinical diagnostic reasoning and diagnostic error. *Journal of Biomedical Informatics, 44*(3), 402–412.

Ma, X., & Hovy, E. (2016). End-to-end sequence labeling via bi-directional lstm-cnns-crf. arXiv preprint arXiv:1603.01354.

McNamara, D. S., Crossley, S. A., & Roscoe, R. (2013). Natural language processing in an intelligent writing strategy tutoring system. *Behavior Research Methods, 45*(2), 499–515.

Naser, S. S. A. (2012). Predicting learners performance using artificial neural networks in linear programming intelligent tutoring system. *International Journal of Artificial Intelligence & Applications, 3*(2), 65.

Nicol, D. (2010). From monologue to dialogue: Improving written feedback processes in mass higher education. *Assessment & Evaluation in Higher Education, 35*(5), 501–517.

Okazaki, N. (2007). *CRFsuite: A fast implementation of conditional random fields*. Retrieved from http://www.Chokkan.Org/software/crfsuite

Papandrea, K., & Winefield, H. (2011). It's not just the squeaky wheels that need the oil: Examining teachers' views on the disparity between referral rates for students with internalizing versus externalizing problems. *School Mental Health, 3*(4), 222–235. https://doi.org/10.1007/s12310-011-9063-8

Reimers, N., & Gurevych, I. (2017). Reporting score distributions makes a difference: Performance study of lstm-networks for sequence tagging. arXiv preprint arXiv:1707.09861.

Reinke, W. M., Stormont, M., Herman, K. C., Puri, R., & Goel, N. (2011). Supporting children's mental health in schools: Teacher perceptions of needs, roles, and barriers. *School Psychology Quarterly, 26*(1), 1.

Rothì, D. M., Leavey, G., & Best, R. (2008). On the front-line: Teachers as active observers of pupils' mental health. *Teaching and Teacher Education, 24*(5), 1217–1231.

Schmidt, H. G., & Rikers, R. M. (2007). How expertise develops in medicine: Knowledge encapsulation and illness script formation. *Medical Education, 41*(12), 1133–1139.

Schrader, F.-W. (2011). Lehrer als Diagnostiker [teachers as diagnosticians]. In *Handbuch der Forschung zum Lehrerberuf* (pp. 683–698).

Schulte-Körne, G. (2016). Mental health problems in a school setting in children and adolescents. *Deutsches Ärzteblatt International, 113*(11), 183.

Schulz, C., Meyer, C. M., & Gurevych, I. (2019). Challenges in the Automatic Analysis of Students' Diagnostic Reasoning. In A. Korhonen, D. Traum, & L. Màrquez (Eds.), The 57th Annual Meeting of the Association for Computational Linguistics - proceedings of the conference: July 28-August 2, 2019, Florence, Italy (pp. 6974–6981). Association for Computational Linguistics.

Simonsohn, A. B., & Fischer, M. R. (2004). Evaluation of a case-based computerized learning program (CASUS) for medical students during their clinical years. *Deutsche Medizinische Wochenschrift, 129*(11), 552–556.

Spinath, B. (2005). Akkuratheit der Einschätzung von Schülermerkmalen durch Lehrer und das Konstrukt der diagnostischen Kompetenz [accuracy of teacher judgments on student characteristics and the construct of diagnostic competence]. *Zeitschrift für Pädagogische Psychologie, 19*(1/2), 85–95.

Trudgen, M., & Lawn, S. (2011). What is the threshold of teachers' recognition and report of concerns about anxiety and depression in students? An exploratory study with teachers of adolescents in regional Australia. *Journal of Psychologists and Counsellors in Schools, 21*(2), 126–141.

Van Merriënboer, J. J., Clark, R. E., & De Croock, M. B. (2002). Blueprints for complex learning: The 4C/ID-model. *Educational Technology Research and Development, 50*(2), 39–61.

Open Access This chapter is licensed under the terms of the Creative Commons Attribution 4.0 International License (http://creativecommons.org/licenses/by/4.0/), which permits use, sharing, adaptation, distribution and reproduction in any medium or format, as long as you give appropriate credit to the original author(s) and the source, provide a link to the Creative Commons license and indicate if changes were made.

The images or other third party material in this chapter are included in the chapter's Creative Commons license, unless indicated otherwise in a credit line to the material. If material is not included in the chapter's Creative Commons license and your intended use is not permitted by statutory regulation or exceeds the permitted use, you will need to obtain permission directly from the copyright holder.

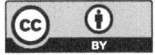

Chapter 9
Live and Video Simulations of Medical History-Taking: Theoretical Background, Design, Development, and Validation of a Learning Environment

Maximilian C. Fink, Victoria Reitmeier, Matthias Siebeck, Frank Fischer, and Martin R. Fischer

This chapter's simulation at a glance

Domain	Medicine
Topic	Dyspnea diseases occurring in an emergency room setting
Learner's task	Take a full medical history in the role of a physician to diagnose patients with dyspnea
Target group	Advanced medical students and early-career physicians
Diagnostic mode	Individual diagnosing
Sources of information	Information is primarily gathered in interaction with the (video) patient. Some prior information (e.g., laboratory and ECG results) is provided by documents
Special features	The content was created for both live and video simulations

9.1 Introduction

History-taking is an essential diagnostic situation for physicians for two reasons. According to a recent literature review, 60–80% of relevant information in medical diagnosing emerges from history-taking (Keifenheim et al., 2015). Moreover, about

---

M. C. Fink (✉) · V. Reitmeier · M. Siebeck · M. R. Fischer
Institute for Medical Education, University Hospital, LMU Munich, Munich, Germany
e-mail: Maximilian.Fink@med.uni-muenchen.de

F. Fischer
Chair of Education and Educational Psychology, Department of Psychology, LMU Munich, Munich, Germany

two-thirds of all medical diagnoses can be made accurately after taking a patient's history (Peterson et al., 1992). Even though history-taking is of such great importance, intermediate students still experience difficulties in conducting comprehensive medical interviews for the purpose of diagnosing (Bachmann et al., 2017). Meta-analytic findings indicate that simulation-based learning conveys diagnostic competences effectively if adequate instructional support is offered to learners (Cook et al., 2010, 2013). Instructional support measures such as reflection phases and role-taking seem promising for fostering diagnostic competences in history-taking situations because they are beneficial for acquiring complex skills in other contexts within medical training (Stegmann et al., 2012; Mamede et al., 2008). Presently, however, only limited empirical findings are available concerning facilitating diagnostic competences in history-taking simulations via these two instructional support measures (Keifenheim et al., 2015). Thus, this project aimed firstly to develop realistic history-taking simulations for the assessment of diagnostic competences. In a second step, this project will use these simulations in future studies that vary reflection phases and role-taking. Dyspnea (shortness of breath) was chosen as the key symptom of the cases in the simulations.

9.2 Theoretical Background

9.2.1 Definition and Models of the Medical Interview

The *medical interview* is a dynamic encounter in which a physician and a patient interactively construct the patient's medical history together (Haidet & Paterniti, 2003). This process is called history-taking. History-taking can be supported with assistive resources (e.g., history-taking forms), and takes place in all medical specialties with direct patient contact in diverse care contexts, including emergency medicine, family medicine and psychiatry (Keifenheim et al., 2015). According to popular models of history-taking (Bird & Cohen-Cole, 1990; Smith et al., 2000; Rosenberg et al., 1997; Kurtz et al., 2003), the medical interview can be conceptualized on a continuum from patient-centered to physician-centered. In patient-centered medical interviews, the patient's psychological and social context is explored more extensively and the patient steers parts of the conversation (Henderson et al., 2012). In physician-centered interviews, by contrast, the patient's physical symptoms are in focus and the physician leads the conversation. The medical interview can perform a wide range of communicative functions, including gathering data and making diagnoses, educating and making decisions, and establishing rapport (Roter & Hall, 1987; Jefferson et al., 2013). Depending on the specific context of a medical interview (e.g., an emergency room vs. a routine checkup), a patient-centered or physician-centered approach with the aforementioned communicative functions might be more relevant (Keifenheim et al., 2015). As this project applies an experimental paradigm and focusses on the simulation-based assessment and training of diagnostic competences in emergency room dyspnea cases, a physician-centered approach emphasizing the functions of gathering data and making diagnoses seems most suitable.

9.2.2 Diagnostic Competences in the Medical Interview

Diagnostic competences have been described on an abstract level using the framework presented in Chap. 2 (Chernikova et al., 2022) and will be specified here in the context of this project.

In all diagnostic settings, diagnostic quality is comprised of diagnostic accuracy and diagnostic efficiency. Diagnostic accuracy generally depends on the correctness of the diagnosis as well as its justification—reasoning for and against the main diagnosis. As it is often not possible to rule out all differential diagnoses in a medical interview without further examinations (Petrusa, 2002), the diagnosis and associated justification may be considered preliminary. Efficiency in history-taking is based not only on time spent, but also on the amount of relevant data gathered in this time and the cost and adverse effects of the examinations and interventions ordered.

The diagnostic process can be operationalized in this context primarily via the diagnostic activities of generating hypotheses, generating and evaluating evidence and drawing conclusions. Hypotheses are frequently formed at the beginning of the medical interview using the patient's background information and initial complaint and are updated over the course of the interview (Pelaccia et al., 2014). Evidence generation takes place in history-taking primarily through asking questions but also includes interpreting visible signs (e.g., paleness as a symptom for pulmonary embolism) and acquiring necessary background information. In the medical interview, evidence evaluation is the analysis of the evidence contained in the background information, the signs and symptoms and the patients' answers. The validity and reliability of the different pieces of evidence can differ significantly and must be determined on a case-by-case basis (Redelmeier et al., 2001). In history-taking, the reliability and validity of evidence can be particularly threatened when information is sensitive or difficult for patients to remember and comprehend. For instance, some patients with extensive medical knowledge present a meticulous documentation of the medication they have taken in the last year in the medical interview, while other patients with low medical knowledge experience difficulties remembering important medication they are currently taking. Drawing conclusions involves weighing the generated and evaluated evidence to make a decision. The result is the creation of a diagnosis and a justification.

According to the theoretical framework presented by this research group, individual prerequisites predict the diagnostic quality and diagnostic process. In the context of the medical interview, the professional knowledge base is a key component of these individual prerequisites (Stark et al., 2011; Förtsch et al., 2018) and can be differentiated into conceptual and strategic knowledge (Schmidmaier et al., 2013; Kopp et al., 2008). Conceptual knowledge is defined as "knowledge about the declarative textbook facts" (Schmidmaier et al., 2013, p. 2), while strategic knowledge "comprises knowledge about problem-solving strategies and heuristics in the process" (Schmidmaier et al., 2013, p. 2). Both types of knowledge, which form the professional knowledge base relevant for the simulation we present in this chapter, include content on diseases that may cause dyspnea as well as content related to conducting the medical interview.

9.2.3 Simulation-Based Learning and Assessment of History-Taking

We propose that history-taking can be facilitated and assessed with live simulations, video simulations and role-plays. Live simulations employ standardized patients who have been systematically trained to act as patients and display symptoms of diseases authentically (May et al., 2009). Video simulations include interactive videos of patients displaying symptoms. User input can take place through a menu or through free text input that is analyzed automatically, e.g., with natural language processing methods (Cook et al., 2010). In role-plays, students receive a script and play the roles of a physician, patient, and observer according to the script (Joyner & Young, 2006). Each of these simulation modalities has certain advantages and disadvantages in medical training. While live simulations are highly interactive, they require a great deal of administrative effort and produce ongoing high costs. Video simulations are expensive at the time of construction but can then be used indefinitely in digital learning environments without new expenditure. Role-plays are inexpensive but require participants to prepare well before taking part.

As seen in Chap. 2 (Chernikova et al., 2022), theoretical arguments and empirical evidence indicate that simulation-based learning with instructional support is a promising method for facilitating diagnostic competences. With regard to simulation-based learning in history-taking situations, 17 studies had been conducted by the time an extensive literature review appeared in 2015 (Keifenheim et al., 2015). Even though most of these studies reported positive effects of educational interventions, the literature review had limitations. Many of the included studies combined numerous educational interventions (e.g., lectures and small group work), focused on communication skills as an output measure or did not include a performance measure of diagnostic competences in the posttest. Specific results for reflection phases and roles are still not available for this context.

Live simulations have been used to assess performance in medicine for decades (e.g., Harden & Gleeson, 1979), and computer-based simulations have become increasingly popular (Ryall et al., 2016). The literature agrees that simulation-based assessment can be reliable and predict clinical performance (Ryall et al., 2016; Petrusa, 2002; Edelstein et al., 2000). However, the reliability and validity of the assessment depend on factors such as the authenticity and standardization of the simulated situation and patient, the choice of scoring algorithms and determination of expert solutions, and the sampling and number of cases (Petrusa, 2002;

Weller et al., 2005; Clauser & Schuwirth, 2002). In general, it is recommended to use multiple, authentic and well-operationalized cases for assessment and to complement simulation-based assessment with other measures such as knowledge tests (Ryall et al., 2016).

9.2.4 Design, Development and Validation Process Objectives and Research Questions

The project focused in this phase on the creation and validation of live simulations and video simulations as assessment instruments. The main research questions were: Are live and video simulations valid and reliable assessment tools? [RQ 1], Are live and video simulations experienced as authentic? [RQ 2], and Are conceptual and strategic knowledge tests predictive of diagnostic quality? [RQ 3].

9.2.5 Simulation Design and Development

The project team consisted of two professors of medicine with expertise in medical education, one professor of educational psychology, a licensed physician and a Ph.D. student in learning sciences. The physician was mainly responsible for creating the content of the simulations and knowledge tests. The Ph.D. student primarily had the task of designing and conducting the experimental study. The professors acquired funding, supervised the physician and the Ph.D. student and offered feedback and advice on their academic work.

In a first step, dyspnea, the subjective feeling of shortness of breath, was selected as a cardinal symptom because it is one of the most common presentations in emergency rooms and GP practices (Berliner et al., 2016). A blueprint was drafted that specified the diagnoses of three training and six assessment cases. Two of the training cases focused on cardiac insufficiency and pulmonary embolism, while for one training case the diagnosis was COPD. Four of the six assessment cases involved specific types of cardiac insufficiency and pulmonary embolism (near transfer), while for two cases the diagnoses were hyperventilation and pneumonia, which are not similar to any training case (far transfer). Next, a case scenario was created to determine the structure and sequence of all cases. All cases would start with key prior information (such as a pathological laboratory test result or an ECG) and a presentation of the chief complaint by the patient. Then, the cases would proceed and be followed by 8 min of history-taking during which the participant could ask or select questions independently. In this phase, participants would mainly conduct a physician-centered interview, asking or selecting general screening questions (e.g., "Is this the first time you are encountering this problem?") and specific questions to test certain diagnoses (e.g., "Have you had swollen legs?"). The

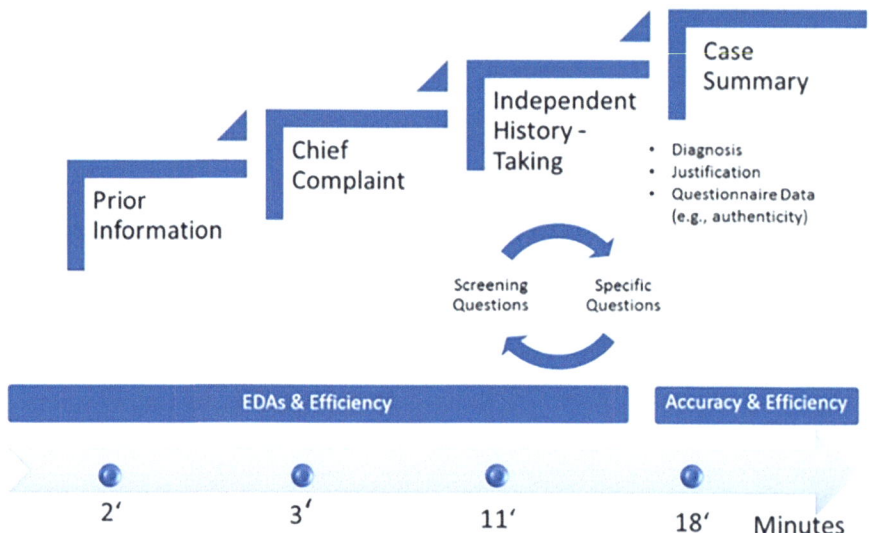

Fig. 9.1 Simulation scenario

questions covered the history-taking categories of principal symptoms, past medical history, allergies and current medication, social and family history and system overview and were based on a classification by Bornemann (2016). Then, students would provide a diagnosis and a justification in a case summary. Figure 9.1 depicts the simulation scenario, including the length of its elements and relevant processes (for more information, see the next section).

Developing a foundation for the live and video simulations, the licensed physician first created a set of history-taking questions as well as nine case vignettes. To create video simulations, a computer scientist programmed a video simulator with a menu and integrated it into the e-learning platform CASUS 3.0 (Instruct, 2018). Professional actors were filmed acting out the cases as standardized patients in a clinical setting and the videos were cut and embedded in the simulator. To produce live simulations, an experimental protocol was created that outlined the behavior of standardized patients and experimenters. The actors were trained to act out the case in face-to-face encounters and individual coaching was offered by the licensed physician. The simulations were conducted in a simulation center at the University Hospital of LMU Munich in Germany that offered three test rooms with a stretcher for the live simulations as well as a computer room for the video simulations and pretest. The final live simulation is displayed in Fig. 9.2 and the final video simulation in Fig. 9.3.

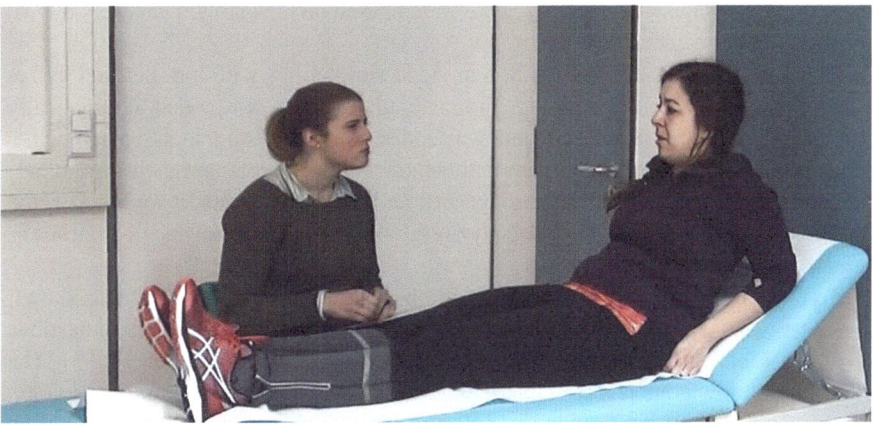

Fig. 9.2 Live Simulation of History-taking

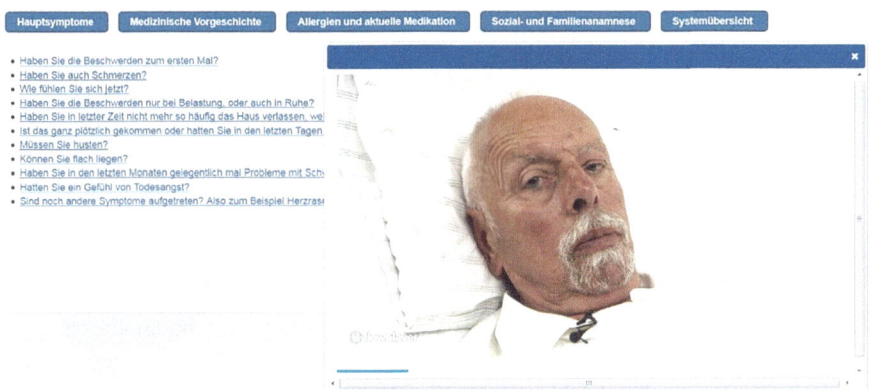

Fig. 9.3 Video Simulation of History-taking

9.2.6 Test Design and Development

To measure diagnostic competences according to the framework described in Chap. 2, separate measures for diagnostic quality, the diagnostic process and the professional knowledge base were created.

Diagnostic quality was assessed with a case summary after each case. Participants listed the final diagnosis in the case summary and provided a justification for this diagnosis. Moreover, participants listed further examinations and treatments. The final diagnosis was chosen from a long menu (i.e., an auto-complete search list that contained many possible diagnoses) and the justifications, examinations and treatments were entered in a text field. Diagnostic accuracy was calculated by adding up partial scores for the final diagnosis (incorrect vs. partially correct vs. correct). The justification for the diagnosis was determined by the percentage of correct reasons mentioned out of all correct reasons for a case defined in the expert solution. Both of these facets of diagnostic accuracy were coded based on the learners' answers by two physicians with a scoring rubric.

Diagnostic processes were tracked in video simulations with log files and in live simulations with video recordings. Video simulation data was coded automatically using *R* scripts. Live simulation data was coded by trained student assistants with a scoring rubric. In both types of simulations, tracked behaviors and their timestamps facilitated detailed analyses of the diagnostic activities. For instance, we investigated evidence generation in depth by analyzing the number and relevance of questions selected.

To measure the professional knowledge base, a conceptual and strategic knowledge test was created. These knowledge tests were based on the conceptualizations of professional knowledge by Förtsch et al. (2018) and Fischer et al. (2005). The conceptual knowledge test contained 39 questions and covered symptoms, etiology, therapy and further diagnostics and interventions for dyspnea. The questions used were extracted from a professional database for examinations. This knowledge test encompassed multiple-choice questions with a varying number of correct answers. The strategic knowledge test consisted of 10 key feature cases (i.e., short case vignettes that contain crucial clinical problems, see Hrynchak et al., 2014) on the topic of dyspnea that were developed by the physician as part of the project. Each case vignette contained four questions on the diagnosis, history-taking, treatment and further diagnosis.

9.2.7 Cooperation with Other Projects

The materials presented above were developed in collaboration with another project on facilitating cooperative medical diagnosing competences (Radkowitsch et al., 2022). Both projects developed comparable simulation blueprints and used the same case summary. The strategic and conceptual knowledge tests were structured in a similar way. Close collaboration also took place with yet another project on diagnostic competences in the diagnostic interview in mathematics education (Marczynski et al., 2022). This collaboration was mainly related to creating the live simulation. In both projects, similar blueprints were created before writing the case vignettes. Standardized patients and students were trained comparably. Measures of diagnostic accuracy and diagnostic processes were operationalized in a similar way in both projects.

9.2.8 Validation Process

A pilot study, an expert workshop and a validation study were conducted to evaluate topics such as the usability, authenticity and correctness of the simulations and tests and to make revisions.

A sample of $N = 12$ medical students took part in the pilot study. The video simulation in the pilot study involved a prototype of the video simulator programmed by the first author and the live simulation employed trained student assistants as actors. Participants diagnosed one case in the video simulation and one case in the live simulation; the sequence of the simulations was randomized. Initial results of the pilot study showed that participants displayed slightly higher diagnostic accuracy in video simulations than in live simulations, and that live simulations were perceived as more authentic than video simulations (Fink et al., 2018). Because of technical problems with the video simulation, a computer scientist produced a professionally programmed video simulation for the validation study. It also became evident that non-professional actors in the live simulation did not act in a highly standardized and authentic way. Therefore, professional actors with experience as standardized patients rather than student assistants were trained to act in the live simulation for the validation study.

To evaluate the authenticity and difficulty of the nine developed case vignettes, an expert workshop with $N = 8$ licensed physicians was conducted. The physicians judged seven case vignettes as authentic and of adequate difficulty for the study and suggested major revisions to two cases. Modifications were made accordingly before all scripts for the video simulation were filmed and before actors prepared for the live simulation.

A total of $N = 86$ medical students took part in the validation study. The study used a mixed design with the between factor expertise (novices vs. interns) and the within factor sequence (video simulations—live simulations vs. live simulations—video simulations). Participants were eligible if they were either in the first 2 years of the clinical part of their university education (novices) or in their final clinical year (interns). Moreover, participants had to be fluent in German to rule out possible effects of language competence. The study used the final live and video simulations presented in this chapter. Participants were randomly assigned to one of the two sequences and took part in a pretest of conceptual and strategic knowledge and then solved three cases in each sequence. Initial findings indicate higher diagnostic accuracy of student participants in live than in video simulations (Fink et al., 2019). These findings are opposed to the findings of the pilot study. Due to the revised simulations, the larger sample, and the higher number of cases, the results of the validation study seem more reliable. Moreover, similarly to the pilot study, live simulations were perceived as more authentic than video simulations. The created knowledge tests were reliable and differentiated between novices and interns. In correlational analyses of the validity of the different knowledge tests and simulations, strategic and conceptual knowledge correlated positively with diagnostic performance in the simulations. Both types of knowledge correlated positively with each other.

All in all, the reported findings demonstrate that live simulations are suitable for the reliable and valid assessment of diagnostic competences in history-taking and offer even higher interactivity and authenticity than video simulations. The created video simulations may still require certain changes, such as longer familiarization with the history-taking menu, to achieve comparable validity and reliability to live simulations and may then be suitable for the economical and standardized assessment of medical interviewing skills. The validity and reliability of the developed knowledge tests were confirmed.

9.2.9 Conclusion Summary

This chapter reported on the theoretical background and the design, development, and validation process of a research project investigating the facilitation of diagnostic competences in live and video history-taking simulations.

In the section on the theoretical background, the summarized models of history-taking showed that a physician-centered approach to history-taking that emphasizes the functions of gathering data and making diagnoses is suitable for the assessment of diagnostic competences in experimental settings. Moreover, the section on diagnostic competences in the medical interview adapted the conceptual model presented in Chap. 2 to history-taking by presenting sensible operationalizations of diagnostic accuracy, delineating the major diagnostic activities (i.e., generating hypotheses, generating and evaluating evidence and drawing conclusions), and specifying the topics relevant for the assessment of professional knowledge in this situation. In addition, possible benefits and drawbacks of live simulations, video simulations and role-plays were outlined. The summary of key findings on training and assessing history-taking with simulations demonstrated that the differential effects of role-taking and reflection phases need further research.

The section on the design, development, and validation process highlighted the importance of systematic design, expert workshops, pilot studies and validation studies. It contains materials and operationalizations for future studies and programs seeking to design interactive history-taking simulations. The presented materials also show how comparable live and video simulations can be designed and developed. Findings from the validation study suggest that the created simulations may be employed after making minor changes, and the knowledge tests assess separate but related aspects of diagnostic competences validly and reliably.

9.2.10 Open Questions for Research

In line with Question 2 of the overarching research questions mentioned in the introduction by Fischer and Opitz (2022), future studies within this project will investigate the effect of instructional support measures on the acquisition of diagnostic competences. More precisely, the project will examine the effect of reflection phases and role-taking in live and video simulations and role-plays. Even though reflection phases have been shown to be effective instructional support measures (Mamede et al., 2008, 2012; Mann et al., 2009), it is currently not clear whether reflection in video simulations during problem-solving or after problem-solving is more effective and what learning mechanisms, such as the application of certain types of professional knowledge, make reflection phases effective. Another open research question that also contributes to Question 2 of the overarching research questions described in the introduction by Fischer and Opitz (2022) pertains to the effect of roles in live simulations. Learners in live history-taking simulations can learn to take on the roles of a physician, a patient and an observer. While it has been shown that learning in the agent role is effective, there is a scarcity of findings on the patient and observer role (Cook, 2014). As also pointed out for reflection phases, it must be investigated what learning mechanisms arise in different roles. Finally, the effects of roles and reflection phases should also be explored in roleplays. Only a few findings on this topic are available, and these results do not directly relate to diagnostic competences but typically to communication skills (e.g., Lane & Rollnick, 2007).

The project also plans to contribute new findings to the overarching research question 4 mentioned in the introduction by Fischer and Opitz (2022), which addresses how simulations can be adapted to fit learners. We believe an especially interesting question concerns how adaptive scaffolding could facilitate diagnostic competences in video history-taking simulations. One interesting type of adaptive scaffolding to investigate would be the individual selection of cases of suitable typicality for learners. Case typicality denotes the degree to which a certain case corresponds with the prototypical signs and symptoms of a diagnosis (Papa, 2016). Learners could benefit from adapted case typicality by learning on optimally challenging cases in their zone of proximal development, scaffolded by instructional support (Vygotsky, 1978). Another interesting type of scaffolding to examine would be the adaptive use of reflection phases or examples. It is currently not clear whether the meta-analytical finding that examples are more beneficial for novices than reflection phases and reflection phases are more beneficial for advanced learners than examples (Chernikova et al., 2019) can be replicated in an experimental setting. Furthermore, it is unknown how reflection phases and examples interact in simulation-based learning from atypical cases.

Acknowledgments The research presented in this chapter was funded by a grant from the Deutsche Forschungsgemeinschaft (DFG-FOR 2385) to Martin R. Fischer, Frank Fischer, and Matthias Siebeck (FI 720/8-1).

References

Bachmann, C., Roschlaub, S., Harendza, S., Keim, R., & Scherer, M. (2017). Medical students' communication skills in clinical education: Results from a cohort study. *Patient Education and Counseling, 100*, 1874–1881. https://doi.org/10.1016/j.pec.2017.05.030

Berliner, D., Schneider, N., Welte, T., & Bauersachs, J. (2016). The differential diagnosis of dyspnea. *Deutsches Ärzteblatt International, 113*, 834–845. https://doi.org/10.3238/arztebl.2016.0834

Bird, J., & Cohen-Cole, S. A. (1990). The three-function model of the medical interview. In M. S. Hale (Ed.), *Methods in teaching consultation-liaison psychiatry. Advances in psychosomatic medicine* (Vol. 20, pp. 65–88). Karger.

Bornemann, B. (2016). *Dokumentationsbögen der Inneren Medizin und der Chirurgie für Anamnese und körperliche Untersuchung für die studentische Lehre in Deutschland* [documentation forms of internal medicine and surgery for history taking and the physical examination for the medical training of students in Germany: An analysis of content and structure]. Diss. Institut für Didaktik und Ausbildungsforschung in der Medizin der Ludwig-Maximilians-Universität.

Chernikova, O., Heitzmann, N., Fink, M. C., Timothy, V., Seidel, T., & Fischer, F. (2019). Facilitating diagnostic competences in higher education: A meta-analysis in medical and teacher education. *Educational Psychology Review, 32*, 157–196. https://doi.org/10.1007/s10648-019-09492-2

Chernikova, O., Heitzmann, N., Opitz, A., Seidel, T., & Fischer, F. (2022). A theoretical framework for fostering diagnostic competences with simulations. In F. Fischer & A. Opitz (Eds.), *Learning to diagnose with simulations—Examples from teacher education and medical education*. Springer.

Clauser, B. E., & Schuwirth, L. W. T. (2002). The use of computers in assessment. In G. R. Norman, C. P. M. van der Vleuten, & D. I. Newble (Eds.), *International handbook of research in medical education* (pp. 757–792). Springer.

Cook, D. A. (2014). How much evidence does it take? A cumulative meta-analysis of outcomes of simulation-based education. *Medical Education, 48*, 750–760. https://doi.org/10.1111/medu.12473

Cook, D. A., Erwin, P. J., & Triola, M. M. (2010). Computerized virtual patients in health professions education: A systematic review and meta-analysis. *Academic Medicine, 85*, 1589–1602. https://doi.org/10.1097/ACM.0b013e3181edfe13

Cook, D. A., Hamstra, S. J., Brydges, R., Zendejas, B., Szostek, J. H., Wang, A. T., et al. (2013). Comparative effectiveness of instructional design features in simulation-based education: Systematic review and meta-analysis. *Medical Teacher, 35*, e867–e898. https://doi.org/10.3109/0142159X.2012.714886

Edelstein, R. A., Reid, H. M., Usatine, R., & Wilkes, M. S. (2000). A comparative study of measures to evaluate medical students' performances. *Academic Medicine, 75*, 825–833. https://doi.org/10.1097/00001888-200008000-00016

Fink, M. C., Fischer, F., Siebeck, M., Gerstenkorn, H., & Fischer, M. R. (2018). Diagnoseakkuratheit und Authentizität in live- und Videosimulationen von Anamnesegesprächen: Ergebnisse einer Pilotstudie [diagnostic accuracy and authenticity of live and video simulations of history taking: Results of a pilot study]. In *Paper presented at the Jahrestagung der Gesellschaft für Medizinische Ausbildung (GMA), Wien, September, 19*.

Fink, M. C., Siebeck, M., Fischer, F., & Fischer, M. R. (2019). Assessing diagnostic competencies with standardized patients and interactive video simulations: Results from a study on history taking. In *Paper presented at the RIME 2019, Copenhagen, May 24*.

Fischer, M. R., Kopp, V., Holzer, M., Ruderich, F., & Junger, J. (2005). A modified electronic key feature examination for undergraduate medical students: Validation threats and opportunities. *Medical Teacher, 27*, 450–455. https://doi.org/10.1080/01421590500078471

Förtsch, C., Sommerhoff, D., Fischer, F., Fischer, M. R., Girwidz, R., Obersteiner, A., et al. (2018). Systematizing professional knowledge of medical doctors and teachers: Development of an interdisciplinary framework in the context of diagnostic competences. *Educational Sciences, 8*, 207. https://doi.org/10.3390/educsci8040207

Haidet, P., & Paterniti, D. A. (2003). "Building" a history rather than "taking" one: A perspective on information sharing during the medical interview. *Archives of Internal Medicine, 163*, 1134–1140. https://doi.org/10.1001/archinte.163.10.1134

Harden, R. M., & Gleeson, F. A. (1979). Assessment of clinical competence using an objective structured clinical examination (OSCE). *Medical Education, 13*, 39–54. https://doi.org/10.1111/j.1365-2923.1979.tb00918.x

Henderson, M. R., Tierney, L. M., & Smetana, G. W. (Eds.). (2012). *The patient history: An evidence-based approach to differential diagnosis* (2nd ed.). McGraw-Hill.

Hrynchak, P., Glover Takahashi, S., & Nayer, M. (2014). Key-feature questions for assessment of clinical reasoning: A literature review. *Medical Education, 48*, 870–883. https://doi.org/10.1111/medu.12509

Instruct. (2018). *Casus [Computer software]: E-teaching and e-learning software for virtual patients*. https://www.instruct.eu/casus/virtual-patients-software

Jefferson, L., Bloor, K., Birks, Y., Hewitt, C., & Bland, M. (2013). Effect of physicians' gender on communication and consultation length: A systematic review and meta-analysis. *Journal of Health Services Research & Policy, 18*, 242–248. https://doi.org/10.1177/1355819613486465

Joyner, B., & Young, L. (2006). Teaching medical students using role play: Twelve tips for successful role plays. *Medical Teacher, 28*, 225–229. https://doi.org/10.1080/01421590600711252

Keifenheim, K. E., Teufel, M., Ip, J., Speiser, N., Leehr, E. J., Zipfel, S., et al. (2015). Teaching history taking to medical students: A systematic review. *BMC Medical Education, 15*, 159. https://doi.org/10.1186/s12909-015-0443-x

Kopp, V., Stark, R., & Fischer, M. R. (2008). Fostering diagnostic knowledge through computer-supported, case-based worked examples: Effects of erroneous examples and feedback. *Medical Education, 42*, 823–829. https://doi.org/10.1111/j.1365-2923.2008.03122.x

Kurtz, S., Silverman, J., Benson, J., & Draper, J. (2003). Marrying content and process in clinical method teaching: Enhancing the Calgary-Cambridge guides. *Academic Medicine, 78*(8), 802–809.

Lane, C., & Rollnick, S. (2007). The use of simulated patients and role-play in communication skills training: A review of the literature to august 2005. *Patient Education and Counseling, 67*, 13–20. https://doi.org/10.1016/j.pec.2007.02.011

Mamede, S., Schmidt, H. G., & Penaforte, J. C. (2008). Effects of reflective practice on the accuracy of medical diagnoses. *Medical Education, 42*, 468–475. https://doi.org/10.1111/j.1365-2923.2008.03030.x

Mamede, S., van Gog, T., Moura, A. S., de Faria, R. M. D., Peixoto, J. M., Rikers, R. M. J. P., et al. (2012). Reflection as a strategy to foster medical students' acquisition of diagnostic competence. *Medical Education, 46*, 464–472. https://doi.org/10.1111/j.1365-2923.2012.04217.x

Mann, K., Gordon, J., & MacLeod, A. (2009). Reflection and reflective practice in health professions education: A systematic review. *Advances in Health Sciences Education, 14*, 595–621. https://doi.org/10.1007/s10459-007-9090-2

Marczynski, B., Kaltefleiter, L. J., Siebeck, M., Wecker, C., Stürmer, K., & Ufer, S. (2022). Diagnosing 6h Graders' understanding of decimal fractions—fostering mathematics pre-service Teachers' diagnostic competences with simulated one-to-one interviews. In F. Fischer & A. Opitz (Eds.), *Learning to diagnose with simulations—Examples from teacher education and medical education*. Springer.

May, W., Park, J. H., & Lee, J. P. (2009). A ten-year review of the literature on the use of standardized patients in teaching and learning: 1996–2005. *Medical Teacher, 31*, 487–492. https://doi.org/10.1080/01421590802530898

Papa, F. J. (2016). A dual processing theory based approach to instruction and assessment of diagnostic competencies. *Medical Science Educator, 26*, 787–795. https://doi.org/10.1007/s40670-016-0326-8

Pelaccia, T., Tardif, J., Triby, E., Ammirati, C., Bertrand, C., Dory, V., et al. (2014). How and when do expert emergency physicians generate and evaluate diagnostic hypotheses? A qualitative study using head-mounted video cued-recall interviews. *Annals of Emergency Medicine, 64*, 575–585. https://doi.org/10.1016/j.annemergmed.2014.05.003

Peterson, M. C., Holbrook, J. H., Hales, D., & Smith, N. L. (1992). Contributions of the history, physical examination, and laboratory investigation in making medical diagnoses. *Western Journal of Medicine, 156*(2), 163–165.

Petrusa, E. R. (2002). Clinical performance assessments. In G. R. Norman, C. P. M. van der Vleuten, & D. I. Newble (Eds.), *International handbook of research in medical education* (pp. 673–709). Springer.

Radkowitsch, A., Sailer, M., Fischer, M. R., Schmidmaier, R., & Fischer, F. (2022). Learning collaborative diagnosing in medical education—Diagnosing a patient's disease in collaboration with a simulated radiologist. In F. Fischer & A. Opitz (Eds.), *Learning to diagnose with simulations—Examples from teacher education and medical education*. Springer.

Redelmeier, D. A., Tu, J. V., Schull, M. J., Ferris, L. E., & Hux, J. E. (2001). Problems for clinical judgement: 2. Obtaining a reliable past medical history. *Canadian Medical Association Journal, 164*(6), 809–813.

Rosenberg, E. E., Lussier, M.-T., & Beaudoin, C. (1997). Lessons for clinicians from physician-patient communication literature. *Journal of the American Medical Association, 6*(3), 279–283.

Roter, D. L., & Hall, J. A. (1987). Physicians' interviewing styles and medical information obtained from patients. *Journal of General Internal Medicine, 2*, 325–329. https://doi.org/10.1007/BF02596168

Ryall, T., Judd, B. K., & Gordon, C. J. (2016). Simulation-based assessments in health professional education: A systematic review. *Journal of Multidisciplinary Healthcare, 9*, 69–82. https://doi.org/10.2147/JMDH.S92695

Schmidmaier, R., Eiber, S., Ebersbach, R., Schiller, M., Hege, I., Holzer, M., et al. (2013). Learning the facts in medical school is not enough: Which factors predict successful application of procedural knowledge in a laboratory setting? *BMC Medical Education, 13*, 722. https://doi.org/10.1186/1472-6920-13-28

Smith, R. C., Marshall-Dorsey, A. A., Osborn, G. G., Shebroe, V., Lyles, J. S., Stoffelmayr, B. E., et al. (2000). Evidence-based guidelines for teaching patient-centered interviewing. *Patient Education and Counseling, 39*(1), 27–36.

Stark, R., Kopp, V., & Fischer, M. R. (2011). Case-based learning with worked examples in complex domains: Two experimental studies in undergraduate medical education. *Learning and Instruction, 21*, 22–33. https://doi.org/10.1016/j.learninstruc.2009.10.001

Stegmann, K., Pilz, F., Siebeck, M., & Fischer, F. (2012). Vicarious learning during simulations: Is it more effective than hands-on training? *Medical Education, 46*, 1001–1008. https://doi.org/10.1111/j.1365-2923.2012.04344.x

Vygotsky, L. (1978). Interaction between learning and development. In M. Gauvin & M. Cole (Eds.), *Readings on the development of children* (pp. 34–40). Scientific American Books.

Weller, J. M., Robinson, B. J., Jolly, B., Watterson, L. M., Joseph, M., Bajenov, S., et al. (2005). Psychometric characteristics of simulation-based assessment in anaesthesia and accuracy of self-assessed scores. *Anaesthesia, 60*, 245–250. https://doi.org/10.1111/j.1365-2044.2004.04073.x

Open Access This chapter is licensed under the terms of the Creative Commons Attribution 4.0 International License (http://creativecommons.org/licenses/by/4.0/), which permits use, sharing, adaptation, distribution and reproduction in any medium or format, as long as you give appropriate credit to the original author(s) and the source, provide a link to the Creative Commons license and indicate if changes were made.

The images or other third party material in this chapter are included in the chapter's Creative Commons license, unless indicated otherwise in a credit line to the material. If material is not included in the chapter's Creative Commons license and your intended use is not permitted by statutory regulation or exceeds the permitted use, you will need to obtain permission directly from the copyright holder.

Chapter 10
Diagnosing Collaboratively: A Theoretical Model and a Simulation-Based Learning Environment

Anika Radkowitsch, Michael Sailer, Martin R. Fischer, Ralf Schmidmaier, and Frank Fischer

This chapter's simulation at a glance

Domain	Medicine
Topic	Collaboratively diagnosing patients suffering from fever of unknown origin
Learner's task	Taking on the role of an internist to identify likely explanations for the patient's fever and interacting with a simulated radiologist to reduce uncertainty with respect to the assumed explanations
Target group	Advanced medical students and early-career physicians
Diagnostic mode	Collaborative diagnosing by internist and radiologist
Sources of information	Documents (patient's history, laboratory results, etc.); radiological findings that can be requested from a simulated radiologist
Special features	Focus on collaborative diagnostic reasoning; development was based on a model of collaborative diagnostic reasoning (CDR); adaptive and standardized responses from a simulated radiologist (i.e., a computer agent)

A. Radkowitsch (✉) · M. Sailer · F. Fischer
Chair of Education and Educational Psychology, Department of Psychology, LMU Munich, Munich, Germany
e-mail: Radkowitsch@leibniz-ipn.de

M. R. Fischer
Institute for Medical Education, University Hospital, LMU Munich, Munich, Germany

R. Schmidmaier
Institute for Medical Education, University Hospital, LMU Munich, Munich, Germany

Department of Internal Medicine IV, University Hospital, LMU Munich, Munich, Germany

© The Author(s) 2022
F. Fischer, A. Opitz (eds.), *Learning to Diagnose with Simulations*,
https://doi.org/10.1007/978-3-030-89147-3_10

10.1 Introduction

Medical students' diagnostic competences have been investigated mainly as individual competences (Kiesewetter et al., 2017; Norman, 2005). This is not congruent with the daily practice of physicians, as they collaborate with physicians of the same or another specialization on a regular basis (for a definition of collaborative diagnostic competences, see section *Collaborative Diagnostic Competences*). For example, physicians regularly discuss patients' diagnoses and treatment plans in groups. In such so-called consultations, the physicians in charge confer with more specialized physicians to hear their opinions. In roundtables such as tumor boards, several physicians with different specializations discuss and negotiate patient cases to come to an optimal diagnosis or treatment plan for a patient. There is also a need to collaborate with different health care professionals such as nurses (Kiesewetter et al., 2017). Medical educators have recognized the importance of collaborative competences in medical education. For example, the German national competency-based catalogue of learning goals and objectives (NKLM, Nationaler Kompetenz-basierter Lernzielkatalog Medizin) emphasizes the role of physicians as communicators and as members of a team (MFT Medizinischer Fakultätentag der Bundesrepublik Deutschland e. V., 2015). Additionally, several simulation centers at university hospitals such as the one at the University Hospital of LMU Munich have recognized the importance of team trainings (Human simulation center, http://www.human-simulation-center.de/). They offer full-scale trainings of different scenarios with simulated patients, ambulances, and even helicopters. Such simulation-based trainings provide opportunities for practice in a controlled and safe environment. However, full-scale trainings are expensive and time-consuming. Physicians and medical students hence do not actively participate in such trainings regularly and instead spend much time observing peers acting in the simulation (Zottmann et al., 2018). In order to learn complex competences and cognitive skills such as collaborative diagnostic competences, it is necessary that learners practice repeatedly, that they focus on subtasks that are particularly difficult to master (i.e., deliberate practice), and that they reflect on their actions and cognition. In doing so, learners develop internal scripts that guide collaborative practices and, if necessary, modify scripts that do not result in understanding or beneficial actions (Fischer et al., 2013). This project addresses collaborative diagnostic competences and means to assess and facilitate them empirically by introducing the model for collaborative diagnostic reasoning (CDR) and developing a simulation in which medical students can repeatedly interact with a simulated physician.

10.2 Collaborative Diagnostic Competences

To facilitate and assess collaborative diagnostic competences in simulations, it is important to understand the underlying processes of collaborative diagnostic reasoning. Contemporary frameworks conceptualize collaborative problem-solving

(CPS) as an interplay of cognitive and social skills (Graesser et al., 2018). Cognitive skills refer to problem-solving skills that are also necessary for individual problem-solving. For example, in the ACT21S collaborative problem-solving framework, Hesse et al. (2015) suggest task regulation as well as learning and knowledge building as key cognitive skills for collaborative problem-solving. As we are interested in diagnosing, which we consider a specific form of reasoning, we follow the suggestions presented in the introduction by Fischer et al. (2022) to base cognitive skills on eight diagnostic activities (problem identification, questioning, hypothesis generation, artifact construction, evidence generation, evidence evaluation, drawing conclusions, and communicating and scrutinizing; Fischer et al., 2014; Chernikova et al., 2022) that successful diagnosticians need to be able to perform with high quality. However, we go beyond their definition by additionally describing social skills necessary when diagnosing *collaboratively*. Different frameworks (e.g., ATC21S, PISA 2017) identify social skills that differ mainly in their granularity. For example, Liu et al. (2015) suggest four social skills (sharing ideas, negotiating ideas, regulating problem-solving, and maintaining communication) and provide a coding scheme to categorize team talk (Hao et al., 2016). Hesse et al. (2015) propose three main skills (perspective-taking, participation, and social regulation) with two to four subskills each. Particularly in knowledge-rich domains such as medicine, both cognitive and social skills are based on the diagnosticians' professional knowledge base, which consists of conceptual and strategic knowledge (Förtsch et al., 2018). Based on CPS frameworks and diagnostic activities, we define collaborative diagnostic competence as the competence to diagnose a patient's problem by conducting diagnostic activities and by sharing, eliciting, and negotiating evidence and hypotheses and regulating the interaction by recognizing both one's own and the collaboration partner's knowledge and skills. The quality of the diagnosis is defined as its accuracy and efficiency (Chernikova et al., 2022).

While there are a number of models describing the structure of collaborative problem-solving skills (i.e., skills and subskills making up this competence), there is a lack of models describing the processes of collaborative problem-solving (i.e., activities and their reciprocal influences). In this chapter, we propose a process model of *collaborative diagnostic reasoning* (CDR) that is intended to explain the collaborative diagnostic reasoning of two actors (in our example, medical specialists) with respect to a patient case. The model further makes assumptions about the development of collaborative diagnostic reasoning. Thus, the model allows for predictions about the facilitation of collaborative diagnostic reasoning. Below, we describe the CDR model as well as theoretical and empirical findings relevant to it. In addition, we derive empirically testable statements from the model.

10.2.1 CDR Model: Collaborative Diagnostic Reasoning

The CDR model describes a collaborative diagnostic situation in which two diagnosticians with different professional backgrounds collaboratively diagnose patients by generating, evaluating, sharing, eliciting, and negotiating hypotheses and

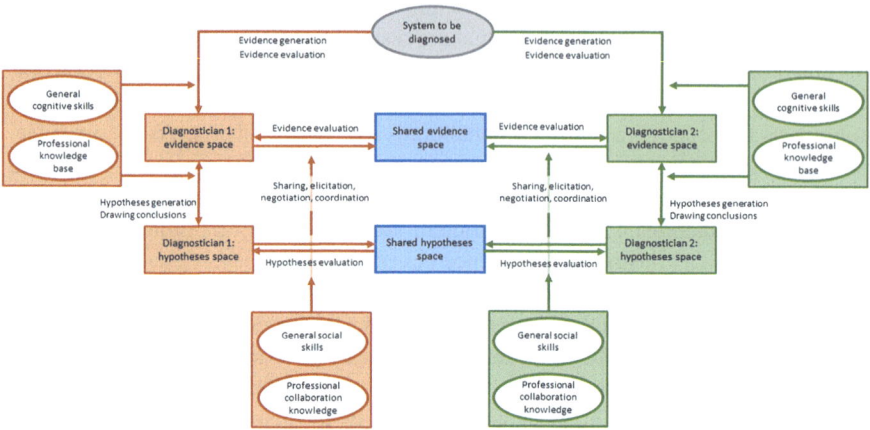

Fig. 10.1 Model for collaborative diagnostic reasoning (CDR) between two diagnosticians. Boxes represent storage areas for outcomes of individual and collaborative processes. Ovals represent individual prerequisites for diagnostic and collaborative activities

evidence. Although the model is introduced here in a medical context, we assume that it is, in principle, also valid for other contexts, such as collaborative diagnostic reasoning among teachers. Although the model in its basic form is limited to two diagnosticians, we do not see any reason limiting the generalization of the model to bigger groups in principle.

The CDR model (see Fig. 10.1) builds on Klahr and Dunbar's (1988) scientific discovery as dual search model (SDDS), but goes beyond it by distinguishing between individual and collaborative cognitive processes. Prior attempts to transfer the SDDS to a collaborative context by Gijlers and de Jong (2005) cannot replace the CDR model, as the extended SDDS describes the structure of individual and shared knowledge but does not identify predictions with respect to individual or collaborative cognitive processes. To describe individual and collaborative cognitive processes, the CDR model builds on the diagnostic activities (generation and evaluation of evidence, generating hypotheses, drawing conclusions) and social activities (sharing, eliciting, negotiating, coordinating) described above. We hereafter term these individual and collaborative diagnostic activities. *Individual diagnostic activities* are conceptualized as the process of coordinating empirical evidence generated by experimenting with hypotheses. Here, we distinguish between a hypotheses space and an evidence space (Klahr & Dunbar, 1988). In the medical context, a diagnostic process is typically triggered by information about the system being diagnosed. The system to be diagnosed is considered to be an external system containing all information about the patient and their social environment that can be considered in the diagnostic process, including, for instance, test results, information about the patients' lifestyle, and symptoms. The diagnosticians start the individual diagnostic process by generating and evaluating evidence. A piece of *evidence* is information on a system with the potential to influence the diagnosis of the system's state by reducing or increasing its likelihood. In the context of medical diagnosing, the evidence typically consists of findings (e.g., laboratory values), enabling conditions (e.g., pre-existing illnesses of family members), and patient symptoms (e.g., stomachache). Evidence is generated by interpreting patient information, sorting out the relevant from the irrelevant information, and generating new information, for example, by conducting a medical test (Fischer et al., 2014). For instance, a radiologist conducts a radiologic test or an internist identifies a patient's lipase laboratory value as abnormally high. Ideally, the generated evidence is evaluated with respect to its validity (e.g., what are the sensitivity and specificity of the test? Are there technical reasons for a false positive value for this test?). Evidence is kept in the evidence space. During the generation and evaluation phases, we assume that participants generate hypotheses and draw conclusions based on the collected evidence (Fischer et al., 2014). A *hypothesis* is a statement about a possible state of the system. The generated hypotheses are stored in the hypotheses space and *tested* in the evidence space by evaluating whether the evidence matches the predictions derived from the hypotheses (Klahr & Dunbar, 1988). By testing hypotheses, diagnosticians draw conclusions which are also stored in the hypotheses space. In our example, the internist who found that a patient has an increased lipase value could generate the hypothesis that the patient suffers from pancreatitis. If the internist finds that the patient additionally suffers from upper abdominal pain (evidence generation), the internist may draw the conclusion that these pieces of evidence speak in favor of the proposed hypothesis.

In collaborative diagnostic situations, physicians additionally engage in collaborative diagnostic activities. In such situations, there is a need to coordinate the evidence and hypotheses space of not one but two professionals. For effective collaboration, it is necessary that the collaborators construct an at least partially shared mental representation of the diagnostic situation (Rochelle & Teasley, 1995). Therefore, we assume that in collaborative diagnostic reasoning, there are two further cognitive spaces in addition to the individual diagnostic spaces: a shared evidence space and a shared hypotheses space. These spaces consist of evidence and hypotheses that are shared among the diagnosticians. All individual diagnostic processes as well as their outcomes (evidence, hypotheses, and conclusions) can become part of one of the shared diagnostic spaces by engaging in the collaborative activities of sharing and elicitation, negotiation, and coordination (Liu et al., 2015; Hesse et al., 2015; Zehner et al., 2019; Mo, 2017). In the literature, the need to share and process information on a group level has been stressed as key to constructing a shared mental representation and successfully collaborating (Hesse et al., 2015; Meier et al., 2007; Larson et al., 1998). The pooling of information allows collaborators to use team members as a resource. Information (i.e., evidence, hypotheses, and conclusions) can be pooled either by eliciting information from the other team member or by externalizing one's own knowledge (Fischer & Mandl, 2003). Negotiating the meaning of evidence and hypotheses are also key for successful diagnosing. The successful negotiation of evidence and hypotheses by two or more diagnosticians can prevent physicians from selecting and interpreting evidence in a way that supports their own beliefs (confirmation bias; Nickerson, 1988; Patel et al.,

2002). Concerning the coordination of collaborative diagnostic reasoning, little research has been conducted. However, findings in the context of collaborative learning underline the importance of coordinating goals, motivation, emotions, and strategies in order to successfully solve problems collaboratively (Järvelä & Hadwin, 2013). Finally, before integrating shared evidence and shared hypotheses in the individual reasoning processes, we expect that diagnosticians evaluate the evidence and hypotheses with respect to their validity. Based on shared evidence and hypotheses, the diagnosticians optimally conclude with a diagnosis. In this context, a *diagnosis* is a decision about the most likely current state of a system that is based on data and allows and/or demands concrete diagnostic and/or therapeutic decisions.

The presented model not only describes the collaborative diagnostic process among two diagnosticians, but makes further assumptions about factors influencing the collaborative and individual processes. Below, four factors are introduced, namely the professional knowledge base, professional collaboration knowledge, general cognitive and social skills. We acknowledge that the proposed factors are not exhaustive and that other variables influencing the outcome of (collaborative) diagnosing such as interest (Rotgans & Schmidt, 2014) or personality traits (Pellegrino & Hilton, 2013; Mohammed & Angell, 2003) are missing. Nevertheless, the CDR model is focused on influential factors that directly affect cognitive processes and can be altered by training.

Professional Knowledge Base Professional knowledge, which refers to knowledge about concepts as well as knowledge about strategies and procedures, is important both for competence development (VanLehn, 1996) and for problem-solving (Schmidmaier et al., 2013). Whereas conceptual knowledge refers to knowledge about terms and their relationships (e.g., What are the contraindications for contrast media? What is the physical principle of computed tomography? What is the definition of community-acquired pneumonia?), strategic knowledge refers to knowledge about appropriate strategies and procedures in specific situations (e.g., How can pneumonia be proven radiologically? How can pulmonary embolism be ruled out? How is triple contrast media generated?; Förtsch et al., 2018). Both types of knowledge form the basis for each diagnostician to generate meaningful evidence, correctly evaluate evidence, correctly relate evidence to hypotheses, and draw conclusions. With increasing experience, strategic and conceptual knowledge becomes encapsulated, resulting in a higher diagnostic efficiency compared to novices (encapsulation effect, Schmidt & Boshuizen, 1992).

Professional Collaboration Knowledge Another aspect that has been stressed to influence interaction among problem-solvers is meta-knowledge about the collaboration partner. Meta-knowledge is knowledge about collaboration partners and their disciplinary background, including their goals, measures, and typical priorities. Meta-knowledge is often a result of joint phases in formal education and joint collaborative practices by professionals with different backgrounds (e.g., internists and radiologists). Having a joint basis of professional knowledge is certainly an advantage for collaboration among medical specialists: Findings from the context of collaborative learning suggest that problem-solvers with meta-knowledge about their collaboration partners begin sharing relevant information earlier (Engelmann & Hesse, 2011) and learn more from each other compared to collaboration partners without such meta-knowledge (Kozlov & Große, 2016). However, the literature also suggests that only having meta-knowledge is not sufficient for successful collaboration (Schnaubert & Bodemer, 2019; Dehler et al., 2011; Engelmann & Hesse, 2011). In the script theory of guidance (Fischer et al., 2013), the authors argue that collaborative practices are dynamically shaped by internal collaboration scripts. Internal collaboration scripts consist of four hierarchically ordered types of components (play, scene, scriptlet, and role) that dynamically configure the internal collaboration script to guide the collaborative process. The configuration of the internal collaboration script is influenced by collaboration partners' goals and perceived situational characteristics (Fischer et al., 2013). Hence, whether and how diagnosticians interact with each other depends on their internal collaboration scripts, which are shaped by their prior experience in similar collaborative practices. We consider both functional internal collaboration skills as well as meta-knowledge as important subcomponents of professional collaboration knowledge.

General Cognitive and Social Skills There is much less focus in research on the role of general knowledge and skills that might be applicable across several domains (e.g., complex problem-solving; Hetmanek et al., 2018; Wüstenberg et al., 2012). The evidence seems clear that general cognitive knowledge and skills do not play a major role for the quality of diagnostic activities and the quality of diagnoses (e.g., Norman, 2005). However, their role for early phases of skill development has not been studied systematically in either medical education or research on collaborative problem-solving in knowledge-rich domains (Kiesewetter et al., 2016). It is likely that general cognitive abilities play a certain role in learning and problem-solving, at least in early phases, where collaborators do not have much specific knowledge and experience (Hetmanek et al., 2018). In addition, more general social skills that individuals develop beginning in early childhood, like participation, theory of mind and perspective-taking (Osterhaus et al. 2016, 2017), might play a role during collaborative diagnostic reasoning. Especially in early phases, when more specific meta-knowledge and script components are not accessible or less functional to medical students, it is likely that they try to apply more generic social skills (Fischer et al., 2013).

10.2.2 The Development of Collaborative Diagnostic Reasoning

In the preceding part of this section, the CDR model was used as a descriptive and explanatory model of collaborative diagnostic reasoning and its underlying competences. However, the CDR model also entails assumptions about how the underlying competences develop. These developmental propositions are: (1) The quality of collaborative diagnostic activities and the collaborative diagnoses further improve through multiple encounters with understanding, engaging in and reflecting upon collaborative diagnostic situations (Fischer et al., 2013). (2) Conceptual and strategic knowledge are more closely associated in intermediates and experts as compared to novices, and this is associated with higher diagnostic efficiency in experts and intermediates as compared to novices (*encapsulation effect*, Schmidt & Boshuizen, 1992). (3) Professional collaboration knowledge becomes more differentiated through experience with reflection on collaborative diagnostic situations entailing feedback. (4) The influence of general abilities, knowledge and skills on the quality of diagnostic activities and the quality of the diagnosis are high when professional knowledge on collaboration is low. (5) As professional knowledge becomes increasingly available, the influence of general cognitive skills on diagnostic activities decreases. These developmental propositions are not represented in Fig. 10.1.

10.3 Developing a Simulation to Investigate Collaborative Diagnostic Competences and Their Facilitation

In what follows, we describe the development of a simulation aimed first and foremost at enabling the empirical investigation of collaborative diagnostic competences and their facilitation, building on the CDR model introduced in the preceding section.

Specifying a Medical Context Most literature on collaborative diagnostic reasoning focusses on the sharing of information. As in other contexts as well (e.g., political caucuses, Stasser & Titus, 1985), shared information (i.e., information that is known to all team members) is more likely to be considered in clinical decision-making processes compared to unshared information. This often leads to inaccurate diagnoses and/or treatment decisions (Tschan et al., 2009; Larson et al., 1998). Tschan et al. (2009) call the unsuccessful exchange of information an illusory transactive memory system, because team members act as if the information exchange was functioning well. Apparently, information exchange seems to be particularly negatively influenced during times of high workloads (Mackintosh et al., 2009). Kripalani et al. (2007) conducted a systematic review of the quality of information exchange between hospital-based and primary care physicians. The authors rated the general information exchange as rather poor. In most of the analyzed articles, important information such as diagnostic test results, discharge medications, treatment course data, or follow-up plans were reported to be missing. Also, health care professionals interviewed by Suter et al. (2009) agreed that information was often not conveyed appropriately for the intended audience. Nevertheless, it seems that it is the relevance and quality of the shared information rather than the quantity that affects the quality of the diagnosis. There is no evidence that the quality of diagnoses increases when more information is shared among team members (Kiesewetter et al., 2017; Tschan et al., 2009). To simulate collaborative diagnostic competences, we first chose a collaborative situation between internists and radiologists as the simulation context. This decision was made based on practitioners' experiences that these two professions interact regularly in the hospital. Afterwards, we conducted interviews with seven practitioners from both disciplines to identify a specific situation that is considered problematic. The interviews revealed that the main problem is suboptimal quality of requests from clinicians for radiological imaging (i.e., elicitation of new evidence from a collaboration partner). A main issue here is unprecise justifications for the examination (e.g., missing relevant patient information) and a lack of clustering of patient information (i.e., low-quality sharing of evidence and hypotheses). These findings are in line with prior empirical findings on sharing skills and suggest that being able to conduct collaborative activities, in particular sharing and eliciting evidence and hypotheses, is particularly important in this specific situation (Davies et al., 2018). Therefore, we decided to focus on the collaborative diagnostic activities of sharing and elicitation. Additionally, we analyzed and compared different learning platforms in order to identify the most suitable platform. We chose the learning platform CASUS (https://www.instruct.eu/) as this platform is suitable for case-based learning and medical students at many universities across the globe are familiar with it.

Design and Development There are different ways to assess and simulate collaborative processes. Traditionally, a team or group of learners is confronted with a problem or patient, respectively (Hesse et al., 2015; Rummel & Spada, 2005). However, there are several issues that go along with this type of simulation. A main issue is that in such situations, the collaboration is influenced by variables such as personality, group constellation, or motivation (Graesser et al., 2018). This makes it more difficult to assess collaborative competences, as the assessments might be confounded. With respect to facilitating collaborative competences, simulations allow learners to deliberately practice subtasks repeatedly in order to improve the quality of specific activities. This is hardly possible during collaboration with real collaboration partners. A more recent approach that might provide a remedy is to use simulated agents (i.e., computer-simulated persons) as collaboration partners (e.g., Mo, 2017). The use of computer agents addresses the aforementioned issues, as the collaboration partners are standardized and hence, the assessment is not affected by variables such as group constellation, personality, or motivation. In this form, the collaboration is of course less flexible (e.g., less conditional branching) but easier to evaluate. Furthermore, a simulated collaboration partner is patient with respect to errors and repetitions and can easily be adjusted to the learners' needs to increase training effects. After we had defined the context of the simulation and decided to use a simulated agent, we developed a schematic representation of the diagnostic situation based on the conducted interviews and further discussions with experts from internal medicine and radiology. The schematic representation (see Fig. 10.2) constrained the storyboard of the simulation and included information about the simulation procedure and possibilities to interact with the simulated radiologist in different ways. The schema was discussed and refined in discussions with experts from medicine, psychology, and software development. During this process, we further decided to construct a document based simulation since routine interactions

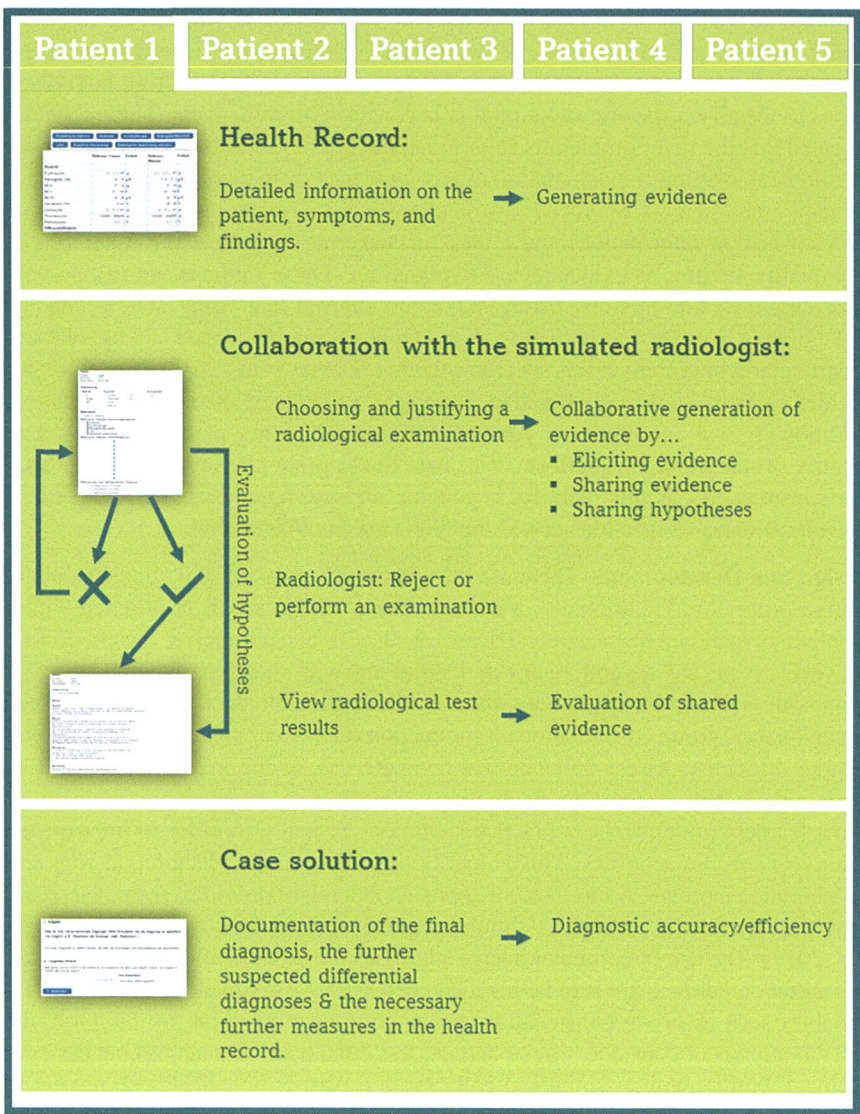

Fig. 10.2 Schematic representation of the simulation: three parts of patient cases (health record, collaboration, case solution)

between internists and radiologists in clinical practice are to a large extent document based. Moreover, this format can also be implemented easily and economically for the training of medical students.

Evaluation The simulation was evaluated twice during its development: once by student participants and once by experts. After completion, a validation study was conducted, which is sketched out below. Firstly, a patient case was developed by two physicians, implemented in the learning platform, and presented to eight medical students in a pilot study. The pilot study aimed at evaluating the simulation's user experience (UEQ, Laugwitz et al., 2008). The results indicated high values on the subscales attractiveness (overall impression of the simulation), perspicuity (simplicity of using the simulation), stimulation (how motivating the simulation is perceived to be), and novelty (degree of innovation), but rather low values on the dependability subscale (perception of control over the simulation). After some adjustments to increase the perceived control, nine additional patient cases were developed by a team consisting of a general practitioner, internists, and radiologists. To do so, complex patient health records and findings from different radiological tests were selected and designed. All health records and radiological findings were structured identically (see Case Part 1: Health record). The radiological findings each consisted of a description of the applied radiological technique, a description of the radiological findings, and an interpretation of these findings. Secondly, to ensure that the cases and their diagnoses were reasonably authentic, all fictitious patient cases were discussed and revised in an expert workshop by experienced practitioners from internal medicine and radiology.

10.4 The Simulation

The developed simulation consists of the familiarization and the fiction contract as well as three sections per patient case, each described in more detail below (see Fig. 10.2). The medical students are first familiarized with the diagnostic situation represented by the simulation by watching a short video. Each patient case is then structured in three parts: medical students first generate, evaluate, and integrate the evidence available in the health records; then they interact with the simulated radiologist to elicit additional evidence; and finally document the diagnostic outcome in the health record.

Familiarization and Fiction Contract At the beginning of the simulation, all participants are introduced to the technical details of the simulation and the diagnostic situation by watching a short video clip. By diagnostic situation, we mean the real-world situation that is represented in the simulation and to which we expect the learners to transfer their knowledge and skills. The learners are informed that they are playing the role of an internist-in-training in a medium-sized hospital and that they will be diagnosing patients' diseases in collaboration with a radiologist. The learners are told that they have seen the patients in the morning and are now revisiting their health records before proceeding with the further diagnostic process. The video clip also clarifies our expectations. For example, learners are reminded that radiological tests are costly, time-intense, and invasive for the patient and that they should try to work as efficiently as possible. In addition, the video clip familiarizes participants with the limitations of the simulation. For instance, the radiologist can only answer priorly defined questions about the radiologic findings (e.g., meaning of specific radiologic terms). We note this explicitly during the introduction in order to avoid confusion.

Case Part 1: Health Record Each patient case starts with a document-based health record containing an introduction to the patient, information from the history-taking, physical examination, laboratory findings, previous diseases, and medication. All cases are structurally equal with respect to the information presented. Learners can take notes while reading the health records. In addition, learners are not interrupted in the first phase of diagnosing. As soon as the learners decide they have collected sufficient evidence to consult with the radiologist, they click the button "request a radiological test." The learners can return to the patient's health record at any time. Log files provide information about the time spent on evidence generation.

Case Part 2: Collaborative Diagnostic Activities Learners in the role of an internist and the simulated radiologist collaborate via a request form and test results. They first elicit the generation of evidence by choosing a radiological test from 42 different combinations of methods and body regions (e.g., cranial CT, chest MRI) and then share relevant evidence (i.e., symptoms and findings) and/or hypotheses (i.e., differential diagnoses). In this way, the learners justify the request and give information relevant to properly conduct and interpret the test results to the radiologist. Specifically, the participants receive a form on which they can tick off symptoms and findings from the health record as well as type in possible diagnoses. The request form allows us to directly measure the quantity and quality of the elicitation of evidence, sharing of evidence and sharing of hypotheses. Only learners who engage in good collaborative diagnostic activities (i.e., appropriately elicit and share evidence and hypotheses) receive the results of the radiological test. Otherwise, the radiologist refuses to conduct the radiological examination and asks the medical student to revise the request form. The result of the radiological test consists of a description of the radiological findings, a short interpretation of the radiological findings, and, only if provided by the learner, an evaluation of the shared hypotheses by the simulated radiologist. As in the health record, we measure the time learners in the role of internist spend evaluating the new radiological evidence. After having read, evaluated, and integrated the results, medical students can ask further questions about the radiological findings to the radiologist by clicking on the respective terms or request additional examinations by the radiologist.

Case Part 3: Diagnostic Outcome To solve the patient case, participants are asked to document the results of their individual and collaborative diagnostic activities in the patient's health record. To do so, they are asked to draw conclusions by suggesting a final diagnosis, backing it up with justifying evidence, suggesting further important differential diagnoses as well as the most important next step in the diagnostic process or treatment. This documentation serves as a basis for assessing the diagnostic quality: Based on the final diagnoses and the provided differential diagnoses, we assess diagnostic accuracy. Diagnostic efficiency is assessed by weighing the diagnostic accuracy against the time needed to solve the patient case (i.e., the more time is needed for an accurate diagnosis, the lower the diagnostic efficiency). After each patient case, learners receive a short sample solution including the most likely diagnosis, the most important findings, as well as differential diagnoses.

In sum, medical students are supposed to first generate, evaluate, and integrate evidence from a patient health record to come up with a hypothesis about the patient's problem and elicit the generation of new evidence in a process of sharing relevant evidence and hypotheses with the simulated radiologist. The newly generated evidence is then integrated with prior evidence to make a final diagnosis. Thus, the simulation allows us to assess and facilitate both collaborative diagnostic activities, namely the elicitation and sharing of evidence and hypotheses, as well as diagnostic quality (i.e., diagnostic accuracy of the final diagnosis and diagnostic efficiency).

10.5 Validation of the Simulation

Before we can use the simulation to validate the CDR model and assess and facilitate collaborative diagnostic competences, we need to test its external validity. We therefore conducted a validation study (Radkowitsch et al., 2020a). Validation is the process of collecting and validating validity evidence with the goal of judging the appropriateness of interpretations of the assessment results (Kane, 2006). We consider the following aspects as evidence for satisfactory validity. Firstly, practitioners in the field rate the simulation and simulated collaboration as authentic (Shavelson, 2012). Secondly, medical students and medical practitioners with high prior knowledge show better collaborative diagnostic activities, higher diagnostic accuracy, higher diagnostic efficiency, and lower intrinsic cognitive load compared to medical students with low prior knowledge (VanLehn, 1996; Sweller, 1994).

We conducted a quasi-experiment in which $N = 98$ medical students with two different levels of prior knowledge as well as internists with at least 3 years of clinical working experience participated. Each participant worked on five patient cases. Experienced internists rated the authenticity of the simulation overall as well as with respect to the collaborative diagnostic process after the second and fifth patient cases. Additionally, we assessed the quality of the collaborative diagnostic activities (sharing and elicitation of evidence and hypotheses), their diagnostic accuracy and efficiency as well as their intrinsic cognitive load.

The results of the study show that the simulation seems to be a sufficiently valid representation of the chosen situation. Internists rated the simulation and collaborative diagnostic processes as rather authentic. Additionally, internists and advanced medical students outperformed medical students with fewer semesters of study with respect to diagnostic efficiency, displayed better sharing and elicitation activities, and reported lower intrinsic cognitive load. Only with respect to diagnostic accuracy did performance not differ across conditions. The reasons for this are probably ceiling effects due to very high solution rates for three of the patient cases—the cases were too easy under the given conditions, so that participants were able to try out a lot of different pathways, repeat the same steps if they wanted to, and share and elicit a multitude of findings and hypotheses with or from the radiologist. However, the diagnostic efficiency clearly demonstrated that experts are better able to solve patient cases within the simulation.

We conclude from our validation study that the evidence for the validity of our simulation is sufficient: we found the expected differences between prior knowledge groups on the most important measures (diagnostic efficiency, sharing and elicitation, intrinsic cognitive load), and the relatively high authenticity rating indicates that the simulation accurately represents collaboration between internists and radiologists. The rather low case difficulty has been increased for upcoming studies.

10.6 Further Questions for Research

Since we found validity evidence for the simulation, our goals for further research are twofold: validating the proposed CDR model and facilitating medical students' collaborative diagnostic competences using scaffolds.

The first goal is to validate the proposed CDR model. As the developed simulation can be considered sufficiently valid, it allows us to test and determine the influence of general cognitive and social skills, professional conceptual and strategic knowledge, as well as professional knowledge regarding collaboration on individual and collaborative diagnostic activities as well as the quality of diagnoses. To validate the CDR model, we propose the following testable predictions based on the description above that will be addressed in upcoming studies: (1) The quality of evidence generation and evidence evaluation depends on strategic and conceptual knowledge and general cognitive skills. (2) The quality of hypothesis generation and drawing conclusions depends on strategic and conceptual knowledge, general cognitive skills, and the quality of the evidence in the evidence space. (3) The quality of sharing, elicitation, negotiation, and coordination depends on professional collaboration knowledge and general social skills. (4) The quality of the evidence in the evidence space depends on the quality of evidence generation and evidence evaluation, the quality of the evidence in the shared evidence space, general cognitive skills, and the professional knowledge base. (5) The quality of the hypotheses in the hypotheses space depends on the quality of hypothesis generation and drawing conclusions, the quality of the hypotheses in the shared hypotheses space, general cognitive skills, and the professional knowledge base. (6) The accuracy of the diagnosis depends on the quality of the evidence in the evidence space and the quality of the hypotheses in the hypotheses space. (7) The quality of shared evidence in the shared evidence space is influenced by the quality of evidence in the individual evidence spaces, the quality of the collaborative diagnostic activities, professional collaboration knowledge, and general social skills. (8) The quality of shared hypotheses in the shared hypotheses space is influenced by the quality of hypotheses in the individual hypotheses spaces, the quality of the collaborative diagnostic activities, professional collaboration knowledge, and general social skills. (9) The influence of professional knowledge on individual and collaborative diagnostic activities is greater than the influence of general cognitive and social skills. (10) The proposed relations are found in different domains in which diagnosticians with different knowledge backgrounds diagnose collaboratively (e.g., teaching).

In the validation study, we not only found validity evidence for the simulation, but also showed that, indeed, medical students with low prior knowledge show low diagnostic efficiency and less advanced collaborative diagnostic activities. This is in line with the reviewed literature (e.g., Tschan et al., 2009) and supports the conclusion that findings from these different medical contexts can be generalized to document-based collaboration in a simulated consultation between an internist and radiologist. Therefore, we seek to address the question under which conditions the simulation can effectively facilitate collaborative diagnostic competences. Sociocognitive scaffolding or external collaboration scripts are instructional techniques that have been shown to have large positive effects on collaboration skills (Radkowitsch et al., 2020b; Vogel et al., 2017). Thus, we are interested in under which conditions external collaboration scripts are effective when learning with simulations. In particular, we examine whether and how adapting collaboration scripts to learners' needs enhances their effectiveness. We assume that adaptive external collaboration scripts could be used to directly scaffold the sharing and elicitation process and thus enhance learners' collaborative diagnostic competences. While external collaboration scripts should have a direct effect on collaboration skills, reflection, a well-analyzed instructional support in medical education (Mamede et al., 2014), should have an indirect effect on the collaborative diagnostic process. The combination of both instructional techniques therefore seems promising for the development of collaborative diagnostic competence, but has not been empirically analyzed yet.

Overall, by addressing these questions, we mainly seek to contribute to Questions 2 and 4 of the overarching research questions mentioned in the introduction by Fischer et al. (2022) and the concluding chapter by Opitz et al. (2022). Moreover, we go beyond these questions by additionally validating the proposed CDR model.

10.7 Conclusion

Collaborative diagnostic competences have been rarely investigated empirically, and little is known about how individual and collaborative diagnostic processes influence each other. We therefore proposed the CDR model to close this gap and to guide further research. To validate the CDR model, we developed a simulation that allows us to assess collaborative diagnostic processes in a standardized environment. As prior findings (Tschan et al., 2009) and the results of interviews we conducted show that medical students and practitioners often have difficulties sharing relevant information, we focused on sharing and elicitation activities during a consultation between internists and radiologists. Through a process analysis, our validation study went beyond just showing that experts perform better than novices. In future research, we will address the question of how using scaffolding with external collaboration scripts and reflection phases facilitates the learning of collaborative diagnostic competences within the simulation. The research that emerges on the use of our simulation and model may also lead to progress in research on collaborative problem-solving (Hesse et al., 2015) and may be transferred to other areas of collaborative problem-solving where learners with different knowledge backgrounds collaborate with each other.

Acknowledgments The research presented in this chapter was funded by a grant from the Deutsche Forschungsgemeinschaft (DFG-FOR 2385) to Frank Fischer, Martin R. Fischer, and Ralf Schmidmaier (FI 792/11-1).

References

Chernikova, O., Heitzmann, N., Opitz, A., Seidel, T., & Fischer, F. (2022). A theoretical framework for fostering diagnostic competences with simulations. In F. Fischer & A. Opitz (Eds.), *Learning to diagnose with simulations—Examples from teacher education and medical education. Springer briefs in education series.* Springer.

Davies, S., George, A., Macallister, A., Barton, H., Youssef, A., Boyle, L., et al. (2018). "It's all in the history": A service evaluation of the quality of radiological requests in acute imaging. *Radiography, 24,* 252–256. https://doi.org/10.1016/j.radi.2018.03.005

Dehler, J., Bodemer, D., Buder, J., & Hesse, F. W. (2011). Guiding knowledge communication in CSCL via group knowledge awareness. *Computers in Human Behavior, 27,* 1068–1078. https://doi.org/10.1016/j.chb.2010.05.018

Engelmann, T., & Hesse, F. W. (2011). Fostering sharing of unshared knowledge by having access to the collaborators' meta-knowledge structures. *Computers in Human Behavior, 27,* 2078–2087. https://doi.org/10.1016/j.chb.2011.06.002

Fischer, F., & Mandl, H. (2003). Being there or being where? Videoconferencing and cooperative learning. In H. van Oostendorp (Ed.), *Cognition in a digital world* (pp. 205–223). Lawrence Erlbaum.

Fischer, F., Kollar, I., Stegmann, K., & Wecker, C. (2013). Toward a script theory of guidance in computer-supported collaborative learning. *Educational Psychologist, 48,* 56–66. https://doi.org/10.1080/00461520.2012.748005

Fischer, F., Kollar, I., Ufer, S., Sodian, B., Hussmann, H., Pekrun, R., et al. (2014). Scientific reasoning and argumentation: Advancing an interdisciplinary research agenda in education. *Frontline Learning Research, 5,* 28–45. https://doi.org/10.14786/flr.v2i3.96

Fischer, F., Chernikova, O., & Opitz, A. (2022). Learning to diagnose with simulations: Introduction. In F. Fischer & A. Opitz (Eds.), *Learning to diagnose with simulations—examples from teacher education and medical education.* Springer.

Förtsch, C., Sommerhoff, D., Fischer, F., Fischer, M. R., Girwidz, R., Obersteiner, A., et al. (2018). Systematizing professional knowledge of medical doctors and teachers: Development of an interdisciplinary framework in the context of diagnostic competences. *Educational Sciences, 8,* 207–224. https://doi.org/10.3390/educsci8040207

Gijlers, H., & de Jong, T. (2005). The relation between prior knowledge and students' collaborative discovery learning processes. *Journal of Research in Science Teaching, 42,* 264–282. https://doi.org/10.1002/tea.20056

Graesser, A., Fiore, S., Greiff, S., Andrews-Todd, J., Foltz, P., & Hesse, F. (2018). Advancing the science of collaborative problem solving. *Psychological Science in the Public Interest: A*

Journal of the American Psychological Society, 19, 59–92. https://doi.org/10.1177/1529100618808244

Hao, J., Liu, L., von Davier, A., Kyllonen, P., & Kitchen, C. (2016). Collaborative problem solving skills versus collaboration outcomes: Findings from statistical analysis and data mining. In T. Barnes, M. Chi, & M. Feng (Eds.), *Proceedings of the 9th International Conference on Educational Data Mining*.

Hesse, F., Care, E., Buder, J., Sassenberg, K., & Griffin, P. (2015). A framework for teachable collaborative problem solving skills. In P. Griffin & E. Care (Eds.), *Assessment and teaching of 21st century skills* (pp. 37–56). Springer.

Hetmanek, A., Engelmann, K., Opitz, A., & Fischer, F. (2018). Beyond intelligence and domain knowledge: Scientific reasoning and argumentation as a set of cross-domain skills. In F. Fischer (Ed.), *Scientific reasoning and argumentation: The roles of domain-specific and domain-general knowledge* (pp. 203–226). Routledge.

Järvelä, S., & Hadwin, A. (2013). New frontiers: Regulating learning in CSCL. *Educational Psychologist, 48*, 25–39. https://doi.org/10.1080/00461520.2012.748006

Kane, M. T. (2006). Validation. In R. L. Brennan (Ed.), *Educational measurement* (pp. 17–64). Praeger.

Kiesewetter, J., Fischer, F., & Fischer, M. R. (2016). Collaboration expertise in medicine—No evidence for cross-domain application from a memory retrieval study. *PLoS One, 11*, e0148754. https://doi.org/10.1371/journal.pone.0148754

Kiesewetter, J., Fischer, F., & Fischer, M. R. (2017). Collaborative clinical reasoning—A systematic review of empirical studies. *Journal of Continuing Education in the Health Professions, 37*, 123–128. https://doi.org/10.1097/CEH.0000000000000158

Klahr, D., & Dunbar, K. (1988). Dual space search during scientific reasoning. *Cognitive Science, 12*, 1–48. https://doi.org/10.1207/s15516709cog1201_1

Kozlov, M. D., & Große, C. S. (2016). Online collaborative learning in dyads: Effects of knowledge distribution and awareness. *Computers in Human Behavior, 59*, 389–401. https://doi.org/10.1016/j.chb.2016.01.043

Kripalani, S., LeFevre, F., Phillips, C. O., Williams, M. V., Basaviah, P., & Baker, D. W. (2007). Deficits in communication and information transfer between hospital-based and primary care physicians: Implications for patient safety and continuity of Care. *JAMA, 297*, 831–840. https://doi.org/10.1001/jama.297.8.831

Larson, J. R., Christensen, C., Franz, T. M., & Abbott, A. S. (1998). Diagnosing groups: The pooling, management, and impact of shared and unshared case information in team-based medical decision making. *Journal of Personality and Social Psychology, 75*, 93–108. https://doi.org/10.1037/0022-3514.75.1.93

Laugwitz, B., Held, T., & Schrepp, M. (2008). Construction and evaluation of a user experience questionnaire. In A. Holzinger (Ed.), *USAB 2008. Lecture notes in computer science* (Vol. 5298). Springer. https://doi.org/10.1007/978-3-540-89350-9_6

Liu, L., Hao, J., von Davier, A., Kyllonen, P., & Zapata-Rivera, D. (2015). A tough nut to crack: Measuring collaborative problem solving. In Y. Rosen, S. Ferrara, & M. Mosharraf (Eds.), *Handbook of research on technology tools for real-world skill development* (pp. 344–359). IGI Global.

Mackintosh, N., Berridge, E.-J., & Freeth, D. (2009). Supporting structures for team situation awareness and decision making: Insights from four delivery suites. *Journal of Evaluation in Clinical Practice, 15*, 46–54. https://doi.org/10.1111/j.1365-2753.2008.00953.x

Mamede, S., van Gog, T., Sampaio, A. M., de Faria, R. M. D., Maria, J. P., & Schmidt, H. G. (2014). How can students' diagnostic competence benefit most from practice with clinical cases? The effect of structured reflection on future diagnosis of the same and novel diseases. *Academic Medicine, 89*, 121–127. https://doi.org/10.1097/ACM.0000000000000076

Meier, A., Spada, H., & Rummel, N. (2007). A rating scheme for assessing the quality of computer-supported collaboration processes. *International Journal of Computer-Supported Collaborative Learning, 2*, 63–86. https://doi.org/10.1007/s11412-006-9005-x

MFT Medizinischer Fakultätentag der Bundesrepublik Deutschland e. V. (2015). *Nationaler Kompetenzbasierter Lernzielkatalog Medizin (NKLM)*. Retrieved from June 11, 2019, from http://www.nklm.de/kataloge/nklm/lernziel/uebersicht.

Mo, J. (2017). How does PISA measure students' ability to collaborate? In *PISA in focus* (Vol. 77). OECD.

Mohammed, S., & Angell, L. C. (2003). Personality heterogeneity in teams. *Small Group Research, 34*, 651–677. https://doi.org/10.1177/1046496403257228

Nickerson, R.-S. (1988). Confirmation bias: A ubiquitous phenomenon in many guises. *Review of General Psychology, 2*, 175–220. https://doi.org/10.1037/1089-2680.2.2.175

Norman, G. (2005). Research in clinical reasoning: Past history and current trends. *Medical Education, 39*, 418–427. https://doi.org/10.1111/j.1365-2929.2005.02127.x

Opitz, A., Fischer, M., Seidel, T., & Fischer, F. (2022). Conclusions and outlook: Toward more systematic research on the use of simulations in higher education. In F. Fischer & A. Opitz (Eds.), *Learning to diagnose with simulations—examples from teacher education and medical education*. Springer.

Osterhaus, C., Koerber, S., & Sodian, B. (2016). Scaling of advanced theory-of-mind tasks. *Child Development, 87*, 1971–1991. https://doi.org/10.1111/cdev.12566

Osterhaus, C., Koerber, S., & Sodian, B. (2017). Scientific thinking in elementary school: Children's social cognition and their epistemological understanding promote experimentation skills. *Developmental Psychology, 53*, 450–462. https://doi.org/10.1037/dev0000260

Patel, V., Kaufman, D., & Arocha, J. (2002). Emerging paradigms of cognition in medical decision-making. *Journal of Biomedical Informatics, 35*, 52–75. https://doi.org/10.1016/S1532-0464(02)00009-6

Pellegrino, J. W., & Hilton, M. L. (2013). *Education for life and work: Developing transferable knowledge and skills in the 21st century*. National Academies Press.

Radkowitsch, A., Fischer, M. R., Schmidmaier, R., & Fischer, F. (2020a). Learning to diagnose collaboratively: Validating a simulation for medical students. *GMS Journal for Medical Education, 37*(5), 2366–5017.

Radkowitsch, A., Vogel, F., & Fischer, F. (2020b). Good for learning, bad for motivation? A meta-analysis on the effects of computer-supported collaboration scripts. *International Journal of Computer-Supported Collaborative Learning, 15*, 5–47. https://doi.org/10.1007/s11412-020-09316-4

Rochelle, J., & Teasley, S. (1995). The construction of shared knowledge in collaborative problem solving. In C. O'Malley (Ed.), *Computer-supported collaborative learning* (Vol. 128, pp. 66–97). Springer.

Rotgans, J. I., & Schmidt, H. G. (2014). Situational interest and learning: Thirst for knowledge. *Learning and Instruction, 32*, 37–50. https://doi.org/10.1016/j.learninstruc.2014.01.002

Rummel, N., & Spada, H. (2005). Learning to collaborate: An instructional approach to promoting collaborative problem solving in computer-mediated settings. *Journal of the Learning Sciences, 14*, 201–241. https://doi.org/10.1207/s15327809jls1402_2

Schmidmaier, R., Eiber, S., Ebersbach, R., Schiller, M., Hege, I., Holzer, M., et al. (2013). Learning the facts in medical school is not enough: Which factors predict successful application of procedural knowledge in a laboratory setting? *BMC Medical Education, 13*, 28. https://doi.org/10.1186/1472-6920-13-28

Schmidt, H. G., & Boshuizen, H. P. A. (1992). Encapsulation of biomedical knowledge. In D. A. Evans & V. L. Patel (Eds.), *Advanced models of cognition for medical training and practice* (Vol. 97, pp. 265–282). Springer.

Schnaubert, L., & Bodemer, D. (2019). Providing different types of group awareness information to guide collaborative learning. *International Journal of Computer-Supported Collaborative Learning, 14*, 7–51. https://doi.org/10.1007/s11412-018-9293-y

Shavelson, R. J. (2012). Assessing business-planning competence using the collegiate learning assessment as a prototype. *Empirical Research in Vocational Education and Training, 4*(1), 77–90.

Stasser, G., & Titus, W. (1985). Pooling of unshared Infomration in group decision making: Biased information sampling during discussion. *Journal of Personality and Social Psychology, 48*(6), 1467–1478.

Suter, E., Arndt, J., Arthur, N., Parboosingh, J., Taylor, E., & Deutschlander, S. (2009). Role understanding and effective communication as core competencies for collaborative practice. *Journal of Interprofessional Care, 23*, 41–51. https://doi.org/10.1080/13561820802338579

Sweller, J. (1994). Cognitive load theory, learning difficulty, and instructional design. *Learning and Instruction, 4*, 295–312. https://doi.org/10.1016/0959-4752(94)90003-5

Tschan, F., Semmer, N. K., Gurtner, A., Bizzari, L., Spychinger, M., Breuer, M., et al. (2009). Explicit reasoning, confirmation bias, and illusory transactive memory. *Small Group Research, 40*, 271–300. https://doi.org/10.1177/1046496409332928

VanLehn, K. (1996). Cognitive skill acquisition. *Annual Review of Psychology, 47*, 513–539. https://doi.org/10.1146/annurev.psych.47.1.513

Vogel, F., Wecker, C., Kollar, I., & Fischer, F. (2017). Socio-cognitive scaffolding with collaboration scripts: A meta-analysis. *Educational Psychology Review, 29*, 477–511. https://doi.org/10.1007/s10648-016-9361-7

Wüstenberg, S., Greiff, S., & Funke, J. (2012). Complex problem solving—More than reasoning? *Intelligence, 40*, 1–14. https://doi.org/10.1016/j.intell.2011.11.003

Zehner, F., Weis, M., Vogel, F., Leutner, D., & Reiss, K. (2019). Kollaboratives Problemlösen in PISA 2015: Deutschland im Fokus. *Zeitschrift für Erziehungswissenschaft, 22*, 617–646. https://doi.org/10.1007/s11618-019-00874-4

Zottmann, J., Dieckmann, P., Taraszow, T., Rall, M., & Fischer, F. (2018). Just watching is not enough: Fostering simulation-based learning with collaboration scripts. *GMS Journal for Medical Education, 35*, 1–18. https://doi.org/10.3205/zma001181

Open Access This chapter is licensed under the terms of the Creative Commons Attribution 4.0 International License (http://creativecommons.org/licenses/by/4.0/), which permits use, sharing, adaptation, distribution and reproduction in any medium or format, as long as you give appropriate credit to the original author(s) and the source, provide a link to the Creative Commons license and indicate if changes were made.

The images or other third party material in this chapter are included in the chapter's Creative Commons license, unless indicated otherwise in a credit line to the material. If material is not included in the chapter's Creative Commons license and your intended use is not permitted by statutory regulation or exceeds the permitted use, you will need to obtain permission directly from the copyright holder.

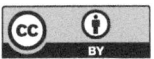

Chapter 11
Conclusions and Outlook: Toward more Systematic Research on the Use of Simulations in Higher Education

Ansgar Opitz, Martin R. Fischer, Tina Seidel, and Frank Fischer

The chapters in this book present a variety of carefully developed simulations of diagnostic tasks. These tasks vary in several key aspects. The learners in these tasks engage in different diagnostic modes and use one of several sources of information. While the simulations in Chaps. 3 through 6 as well as 8 and 9 feature an individual diagnostic process, such as diagnosing mathematical misconceptions, as their diagnostic mode, the simulations presented in Chaps. 7 and 10 require collaboration between two agents, e.g., an internist and a radiologist. In the simulations in Chaps. 3, 8, and 10, learners are required to use documents, such as patients' files or tasks solved by students, to draw a conclusion. In contrast, the simulations in Chaps. 4, 6, and 7 contain videos of critical diagnostic situations such as students constructing an experiment or teachers orchestrating a classroom. A third type of source, featured in the simulations in Chaps. 5 and 9, are standardized live interactions between students or patients.

Additionally, the presented simulations cover various domains and topics. The simulations from the medical domain (Chaps. 9 and 10) address radiological examinations and medical history-taking. Several of the simulations from the domain of teacher education revolve around students' competences and misconceptions, including rather domain-specific competences such as mathematical argumentation

---

A. Opitz (✉) · F. Fischer
Chair of Education and Educational Psychology, Department of Psychology, LMU Munich, Munich, Germany
e-mail: Ansgar.Opitz@psy.lmu.de

M. R. Fischer
Institute for Medical Education, University Hospital, LMU Munich, Munich, Germany

T. Seidel
Friedl Schöller Endowed Chair for Educational Psychology, School of Education, Technical University of Munich (TUM), Munich, Germany

© The Authors(s) 2022
F. Fischer, A. Opitz (eds.), *Learning to Diagnose with Simulations*,
https://doi.org/10.1007/978-3-030-89147-3_11

(see especially Chaps. 3 through 5) but also cross-domain competences such as scientific reasoning (Chap. 7). Other simulations from this domain address topics such as instructional quality (Chap. 6) and learning disorders (Chap. 8).

This diversity is not surprising, as it reflects the variety of real-life diagnostic situations. However, despite these differences, all presented simulations share a common goal: providing students, practitioners, and researchers with tools to test and foster diagnostic competences. Prior studies have shown that it is possible to foster diagnostic competences with a range of learning environments (see a comprehensive meta-analysis by Chernikova et al., 2019). Thus, it is not surprising that several of the simulations presented in this book have already produced promising early results. This is good news for the training of complex skills on the higher education level. However, several research questions remain open at this point. We already mentioned these overarching research questions in the introduction, and the chapters described how they plan to contribute to them. Here, in the conclusion section, we want to provide a more in-depth look at these questions.

11.1 What Processes are Central for Generating Desired Learning Outcomes in Simulations Aimed at Diagnostic Competences?

It is plausible to assume that the improvements that occur in simulations do not happen automatically just by being confronted with a diagnostic task, but because learners engage in certain activities during the diagnostic process. If researchers were better able to describe these activities using a common language across domains, they would be able to conduct coordinated research leading to knowledge accumulation and more efficient learning environments in the future. According to the model presented in Chap. 2 (Chernikova et al., 2022), diagnostic activities are one potential candidate for such a joint language. As simply a common language without an a priori implication for specific sequences of activities, diagnostic activities can serve as the starting point for analyses, especially for processes focused on confirming hypotheses, with activities such as generating hypotheses, generating and evaluating evidence, and drawing conclusions (Fischer et al., 2014). In situations that have a stronger exploratory focus, a different set of activities, such as noticing and knowledge-based reasoning about ongoing observation, might also be a promising conceptualization (Seidel & Stürmer, 2014). In future studies, we not only hope to find out more about the role of diagnostic activities in confirmatory and exploratory diagnostic situations, but also whether this role is different for individual vs. collaborative diagnostic situations, different diagnostic topics, or when different sources of information are used. The diversity of the presented simulations thus proves useful, as it will allow researchers to shed light on these questions.

11.2 How Can Learners in Simulations be Supported in Optimizing Learning Outcomes?

It is known from past research on complex learning environments that learners can become overwhelmed and need additional help if learning outcomes are to be optimized (e.g., Glogger-Frey et al., 2016). This assistance can take various forms, so there is not just one solution to this problem. A rather simple form of assistance can be the additional explicit presentation of information. Having the necessary knowledge base could help learners in the presented simulations focus on the actual diagnostic task-at-hand.

For instance, it might help learners to receive input about common mathematical misconceptions among students or various forms of lung diseases to perform well in diagnosing these entities in the presented cases.

Other promising forms of assistance can be found in the scaffolding literature (Belland et al., 2017; van de Pol et al., 2010). One idea would be to include prompts in the simulations that guide participants' attention to crucial information that is often missed.

Additionally, scaffolding that includes reflection phases could be useful (Mamede & Schmidt, 2017). Stopping the learners' thought process every once in a while and asking them to reflect on whether they are on the correct path might prevent them from drawing premature conclusions and learn more effectively from both their successes and failures in diagnosing.

A third tool would be to let learners take on different roles. Switching from the perspective of the person who conducts the diagnosis to the perspective of an observer or even the patient or student might lead to new insights about diagnostic errors (Stegmann et al., 2012). The presented simulations will not only allow us to see whether explicitly presented information on concepts and procedures as well as scaffolding is helpful, but also which version of this information is most beneficial. It is also important to identify any downsides to additional help, e.g., whether prompts or reflection phases can disrupt learning during the diagnostic process.

11.3 Which Variables Mediate or Moderate the Effects of Instructional Support?

Given that a positive effect of instructional support on learning diagnostic competences in simulations has been found, it would be important to know whether this effect is conditional on other variables. For instance, a potential expertise reversal effect is of interest (Sweller et al., 2003). An expertise reversal effect would mean that beginners benefit from instructional support but more advanced learners might be distracted by the same support features and thus learn less because of them. Furthermore, it should be investigated how important it is that learners feel involved in the simulations and perceive them as authentic. Other variables of interest in this regard include interest, motivation, emotions, and self-efficacy. This set of variables could serve as mediators or moderators of the effect of scaffolding on diagnostic competences. In addition, research should focus on observing the influence of instructional support on learners' cognitive load and whether the effects of instructional support on the learning outcome partly depend on how well a learner has developed basic cognitive functions such as shifting and working memory capacity. All of these variables are known to be important in complex learning environments and thus deserve attention in simulations about diagnostic competences (Glogger-Frey et al., 2016; Miyake & Friedman, 2012; Paas & van Gog, 2006; Pekrun et al., 2016; Renkl, 2014; Rotgans & Schmidt, 2011; Schwaighofer, Bühner, & Fischer, 2017a; Scoresby & Shelton, 2011; Vollmeyer & Rheinberg, 2006; Witmer & Singer, 1998; Zimmerman, 2000).

11.4 How Can the Simulations be Adapted to Fit Learners' Needs?

One question that should be investigated in the future is how the presented simulations can be adapted to the needs of different learners so that the largest possible number of learners will benefit from them. This adaptability comes in various forms and it is possible that simulations will lead to better outcomes if they are designed in a way that can be easily adapted to the needs of different groups of learners or even each individual (Ruiz et al., 2006). One version would be to give different simulations to learners in different stages of the learning process, e.g., beginners vs. advanced learners, which would address the above-mentioned expertise reversal effect. However, it might also be the case that advanced learners benefit from a range of instructional support measures without detrimental effects (Chernikova et al., 2019), so further research should seek to reveal how relevant the expertise reversal effect is in training diagnostic competences with simulations. Adaptability can also occur within a single simulation. The simulation could include a possibility for learners to seek the help they need, which might even lead them to different parts of the same simulation (Kitsantas et al., 2013). Simulations can also adapt themselves, e.g., in the form of adaptive feedback that is specific to the performance of individual learners (Bimba et al., 2017). Additionally, the timing of scaffolding in the course of acquiring diagnostic competences can be adaptive, too. If learners benefit from scaffolding at the beginning but not in later stages of learning, fading scaffolds could be applied (Pea, 2004; Wecker & Fischer, 2011). A related idea is to experiment with the order in which multiple scaffolds are presented to learners, as there are indications in the literature that this can have an influence on learning gains (Schwaighofer, Vogel, et al., 2017b).

11.5 Overview of Future Contributions and their Potential Impact

The simulations described in this book are well-situated to contribute to all of these questions, with the specifics described at the end of the respective chapters. However, to demonstrate the many ways the simulations will help to answer the four overarching research questions, we want to give an illustrative selection of how the projects will address them. Analyses of central diagnostic processes for optimal learning outcomes (Question 1) will be covered, for example, by the simulations from Chaps. 3 and 7 by analyzing learners' notes and the influence of the distribution of information in a collaborative diagnostic process, respectively. The simulation in Chap. 8 tackles Question 2 about support for learners by implementing automated feedback, while the simulation in Chap. 10 will use external collaboration scripts. To find out more about mediating and moderating variables (Question 3), the simulations from Chaps. 4 and 5 will be especially useful. The corresponding projects plan to analyze the effects of variables like interest, self-concept, authenticity and immersion. The fourth and final question about adapting simulations to individual learners' needs will be a focus, for example, for the projects presented in Chaps. 6 and 9. They plan to look at differences between beginners and experienced learners and the influence of the typicality of a case (Papa et al., 1996).

Having the simulations presented throughout this book as tools to answer the questions laid out in this last chapter will not only be important to improve the model of diagnostic reasoning presented in Chap. 2 of this book (Chernikova et al., 2022). These answers are key to ensuring that the highest possible number of learners benefit from the large-scale implementation of simulations as a learning tool for diagnostic competences. One important step in this process is interdisciplinary research, as presented in this book, that brings together experts from different fields and allows researchers to explore whether principles about constructing beneficial simulations transfer across domains. One assumption that can be tested is whether the same principles apply for cognitively similar simulations across domains even if they might not apply for simulations within one domain with different cognitive requirements.

The lessons learned from such an interdisciplinary approach to training diagnostic competences might also be transferable to other relevant higher education skills. The cognitive skills education systems expect higher education graduates to master are complex, and so far ways to test and foster them are scarce (Opitz et al., 2017; Zlatkin-Troitschanskaia et al., 2015). We are confident that the work presented in this book can make a contribution to addressing this problem through interdisciplinary research.

Acknowledgments The research presented in this chapter was funded by a grant from the Deutsche Forschungsgemeinschaft (DFG-FOR 2385).

References

Belland, B. R., Walker, A. E., Kim, N. J., & Lefler, M. (2017). Synthesizing results from empirical research on computer-based scaffolding in STEM education a meta-analysis. *Review of Educational Research, 87*(2), 309–344. 0034654316670999.

Bimba, A. T., Idris, N., Al-Hunaiyyan, A., Mahmud, R. B., & Shuib, N. L. B. M. (2017). Adaptive feedback in computer-based learning environments: A review. *Adaptive Behavior, 25*(5), 217–234. https://doi.org/10.1177/1059712317727590

Chernikova, O., Heitzmann, N., Fink, M. C., Timothy, V., Seidel, T., & Fischer, F. (2019). Facilitating diagnostic competences in higher education - a meta-analysis in medical and teacher education. *Educational Psychology Review, 32*, 1–40. https://doi.org/10.1007/s10648-019-09492-2

Chernikova, O., Heitzmann, N., Opitz, A., Seidel, T., & Fischer, F. (2022). A theoretical framework for fostering diagnostic competences with simulations. In F. Fischer & A. Opitz (Eds.), *Learning to diagnose with simulations - Examples from teacher education and medical education*. Springer. (p. Introduction).

Fischer, F., Kollar, I., Ufer, S., Sodian, B., Hussmann, H., Pekrun, R., ... Eberle, J. (2014). Scientific reasoning and argumentation: Advancing an interdisciplinary research agenda in education. *Frontline Learning Research, 2*(3), 28–45.

Glogger-Frey, I., Gaus, K., & Renkl, A. (2016). Learning from direct instruction: Best prepared by several self-regulated or guided invention activities? *Learning and Instruction*. https://doi.org/10.1016/j.learninstruc.2016.11.002

Kitsantas, A., Dabbagh, N., & Dass, S. (2013). Using learning technologies to support help seeking in higher education contexts. In S. A. Karabenick & M. Puustinen (Eds.), *Advances in help-seeking research and applications: The role of emerging technologies* (pp. 73–97). IAP Information Age Publishing.

Mamede, S., & Schmidt, H. G. (2017). Reflection in medical diagnosis: A literature review. *Health Professions Education, 3*(1), 15–25.

Miyake, A., & Friedman, N. P. (2012). The nature and organization of individual differences in executive functions: Four general conclusions. *Current Directions in Psychological Science, 21*(1), 8–14. https://doi.org/10.1177/0963721411429458

Opitz, A., Heene, M., & Fischer, F. (2017). Measuring scientific reasoning – A review of test instruments. *Educational Research and Evaluation, 23*(3–4), 78–101. https://doi.org/10.1080/13803611.2017.1338586

Paas, F., & van Gog, T. (2006). Optimising worked example instruction: Different ways to increase germane cognitive load. *Learning and Instruction, 16*(2), 87–91. https://doi.org/10.1016/j.learninstruc.2006.02.004

Papa, F. J., Stone, R. C., & Aldrich, D. G. (1996). Further evidence of the relationship between case typicality and diagnostic performance: Implications for medical education. *Academic Medicine, 71*(1), S10. https://doi.org/10.1097/00001888-199601000-00028

Pea, R. D. (2004). The social and technological dimensions of scaffolding and related theoretical concepts for learning, education, and human activity. *Journal of the Learning Sciences, 13*(3), 423–451. https://doi.org/10.1207/s15327809jls1303_6

Pekrun, R., Vogl, E., Muis, K. R., & Sinatra, G. M. (2016). Measuring emotions during epistemic activities: The epistemically-related emotion scales. *Cognition and Emotion*, 1–9. https://doi.org/10.1080/02699931.2016.1204989

Renkl, A. (2014). Toward an instructionally oriented theory of example-based learning. *Cognitive Science, 38*(1), 1–37. https://doi.org/10.1111/cogs.12086

Rotgans, J. I., & Schmidt, H. G. (2011). Situational interest and academic achievement in the active-learning classroom. *Learning and Instruction, 21*(1), 58–67.

Ruiz, J. G., Mintzer, M. J., & Leipzig, R. M. (2006). The impact of E-learning in medical education. *Academic Medicine, 81*(3), 207–212. https://doi.org/10.1097/00001888-200603000-00002

Schwaighofer, M., Bühner, M., & Fischer, F. (2017a). Executive functions in the context of complex learning: Malleable moderators? *Frontline Learning Research, 5*(1), 58–75. https://doi.org/10.14786/flr.v5i1.268

Schwaighofer, M., Vogel, F., Kollar, I., Ufer, S., Strohmaier, A., Terwedow, I., ... Fischer, F. (2017b). How to combine collaboration scripts and heuristic worked examples to foster mathematical argumentation – When working memory matters. *International Journal of Computer-Supported Collaborative Learning, 12*(3), 281–305. https://doi.org/10.1007/s11412-017-9260-z

Scoresby, J., & Shelton, B. E. (2011). Visual perspectives within educational computer games: Effects on presence and flow within virtual immersive learning environments. *Instructional Science, 39*(3), 227–254. https://doi.org/10.1007/s11251-010-9126-5

Seidel, T., & Stürmer, K. (2014). Modeling and measuring the structure of professional vision in preservice teachers. *American Educational Research Journal, 51*(4), 739–771. https://doi.org/10.3102/0002831214531321

Stegmann, K., Pilz, F., Siebeck, M., & Fischer, F. (2012). Vicarious learning during simulations: Is it more effective than hands-on training? *Medical Education, 46*(10), 1001–1008.

Sweller, J., Ayres, P. L., Kalyuga, S., & Chandler, P. (2003). The expertise reversal effect. *Educational Psychologist, 38*(1), 23–31.

van de Pol, J., Volman, M., & Beishuizen, J. (2010). Scaffolding in Teacher–Student Interaction: A Decade of Research. *Educational Psychology Review, 22*(3), 271–296. https://doi.org/10.1007/s10648-010-9127-6

Vollmeyer, R., & Rheinberg, F. (2006). Motivational effects on self-regulated learning with different tasks. *Educational Psychology Review, 18*(3), 239–253. https://doi.org/10.1007/s10648-006-9017-0

Wecker, C., & Fischer, F. (2011). From guided to self-regulated performance of domain-general skills: The role of peer monitoring during the fading of instructional scripts. *Learning and Instruction, 21*(6), 746–756. https://doi.org/10.1016/j.learninstruc.2011.05.001

Witmer, B. G., & Singer, M. J. (1998). Measuring presence in virtual environments: A presence questionnaire. *Presence: Teleoperators and Virtual Environments, 7*(3), 225–240. https://doi.org/10.1162/105474698565686

Zimmerman, B. J. (2000). Self-efficacy: An essential motive to learn. *Contemporary Educational Psychology, 25*(1), 82–91. https://doi.org/10.1006/ceps.1999.1016

Zlatkin-Troitschanskaia, O., Shavelson, R. J., & Kuhn, C. (2015). The international state of research on measurement of competency in higher education. *Studies in Higher Education, 40*(3), 393–411. https://doi.org/10.1080/03075079.2015.1004241

Open Access This chapter is licensed under the terms of the Creative Commons Attribution 4.0 International License (http://creativecommons.org/licenses/by/4.0/), which permits use, sharing, adaptation, distribution and reproduction in any medium or format, as long as you give appropriate credit to the original author(s) and the source, provide a link to the Creative Commons license and indicate if changes were made.

The images or other third party material in this chapter are included in the chapter's Creative Commons license, unless indicated otherwise in a credit line to the material. If material is not included in the chapter's Creative Commons license and your intended use is not permitted by statutory regulation or exceeds the permitted use, you will need to obtain permission directly from the copyright holder.

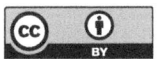

Index

A
Accuracy, 8, 50, 57
Acting training, 56
Adaptability, 146
Adaptive teaching, 18
Agent-based simulation, 131
Approximation of practice
　learning and assessment, 57
　participants' perception, 58
　simulation materials content, 58
　simulation usability, 57, 58
Approximations of practice, 52
Artifact construction, 19
Assessment scenario, 53
Authentic and realistic tasks, 59

B
Bavarian curriculum, 70
Behavioral disorders, 99

C
Case knowledge, 18
Case profiles, 56
Chain of conclusion, 36
Code generating evidence, 74
Cognitive activation, 68
Cognitive functions, 146
Cognitive skills, 124, 125
Cognitive skills education systems, 147
Collaboration, 10
Collaborative diagnostic
　activities, 134, 137
Collaborative diagnostic competences

CDR model (*see* Collaborative
　diagnostic reasoning (CDR))
　cognitive skills, 124, 125
　collaboration scripts, 138
　collaborative problem-solving skills, 125
　CPS frameworks, 125
　diagnostic activities, 125
　internal scripts, 124
　knowledge-rich domains, 125
　medical education, 124
　reflection phases, 138
　simulations, 124
　social skills, 125
Collaborative diagnostic reasoning (CDR)
　cognitive spaces, 127
　collaborative diagnostic activities, 136
　collaborative diagnostic processes, 137
　collaborative diagnostic situations, 127
　collaborative learning, 128
　description, 125
　development, 129, 130
　diagnosis, 128
　diagnostic activities, 126
　evidence is information, 126
　external collaboration scripts, 137
　factors, 128
　general cognitive knowledge, 129
　goal, 136
　hypothesis, 127
　individual diagnostic activities, 126
　individual diagnostic processes, 126, 127
　individual *vs.* collaborative
　　cognitive processes, 126
　information, 127
　internal collaboration scripts, 129

Collaborative diagnostic reasoning (CDR) (*cont.*)
  medical context, 126
  professional collaboration knowledge, 128, 129
  professional knowledge base, 128
  SDDS, 126
  simulation development
    collaborative diagnostic activities, 134
    design, 131
    diagnostic outcome, 134, 135
    evaluation, 132, 133
    familiarization, 133
    fiction contract, 133
    health record, 134
    medical context, 130, 131
    patient cases, 132
    validation, 135, 136
  social activities, 126
  social skills, 129
  studies, 136
  teachers, 126
Collaborative learning, 128
Collaborative problem-solving (CPS), 124, 125, 138
Communication skills, 112
Competence areas, 20
Competence domains, 20
Competences theoretical classification, 20
Complex cognitive skills and competences development, 12
Complex learning environments, 5
Complex practice opportunities, 5
Computer-based simulations, 88
Computer-supported, 98
Concept network, 36
Concept properties, 36
Concept scope, 36
Conceptual framework, 5
Conceptual knowledge, 7, 34, 111, 116, 128
Conceptual model blocks
  context of simulation block, 7
  diagnostic activities, 8
  diagnostic quality, 8
  diagnostic situation nature, 10
  explicit information presentation, 9
  individual learning prerequisites block, 6
  individual learners' characteristics, 8
  instructional support block, 6
  medical and teacher education domains, 11
  processes in simulation-based learning environments block, 6
  professional knowledge base, 7, 8
  scaffolding, 9, 10
  simulations, instructional method, 9
  test performance block, 6
Content knowledge (CK), 7, 18, 20, 34, 51, 65
Content-related prompts, 76
Context of simulation, 7
Cross-domain competences, 144

D

Decimals and diagnosing mathematics skills, 56
Decision-making, 1
Decomposition form, 52
Decomposition of practice, 52
Description, 66
Design of video-based simulation
  diagnostic outcome, 43
  diagnostic process, 42, 43
  diagnostic situation, 40
  diagnostic task, 40, 42
  mathematical argumentation skills, 40
  structure, 40
Diagnosing
  adaptive teaching, 18
  definition, 2
  goal-directed accumulation, 50
  goal-oriented collection, 64
Diagnosing primary student's mathematical competence
  adaptive teaching, 18–19
  operating principle, 24–27
  preliminary findings, 27–28
  simulated environment development, 21–24
  student's solutions, 20
  support, simulated learning environment, 20
Diagnosis, 1
Diagnostic accuracy, 111
Diagnostic activities, 67, 144
  drawing conclusions, 57
  educational settings, 19
  evaluating evidence, 57
  model, 19
  real classroom situations, 20
Diagnostic competences, 85, 86, 98, 100, 101, 104, 111, 112, 116, 118, 124, 144, 146, 147
  definition, 2, 18
  diagnostic activities, 19
  dispositions, 64

indicators, 65
measurement tools, 1
moderator, 12
problem-based learning, 11
problem-solving independent, 12
research, 1
simulation-based learning, 2, 7
teacher education, 50
teachers' individual resources, 50
traditional conceptualization, 58
Diagnostic decisions, 34
Diagnostic demands, 52
Diagnostic efficiency, 9, 134
Diagnostic evidence generation, 57
Diagnostic outcome, 43
Diagnostic problems, 3
Diagnostic process, 8, 43
    commonality, 11
    cycles, 42
    learning environment, 28
    mathematical problem selection, 27
    medicine, 11
    pre-service teachers, 25
    teacher education, 11
    teachers' judgments, 50
Diagnostic product, 57
Diagnostic quality, 8
Diagnostic reasoning, 147
Diagnostic results, 64
Diagnostic sensitivity, 57
Diagnostic situation nature, 10
Diagnostic situations, 34, 40, 50
Diagnostic skills, 34, 44
Diagnostic task, 40, 42, 55
Diagnosticians, 2
Digital learning environments, 98
Digital simulations, 6
DiKoBi
    classroom situations, 67
    data generation, 72, 74
    diagnosing effective teaching, 76
    diagnostic competences use, 69
    interdisciplinary collaboration, 76
    research questions, 69
    simulation and diagnostic process, 71, 72
    situation-specific skills measurement, 69
    specific classroom situations, 70
    university courses, 76
    validation, 74, 75
    video-based simulation, 64, 70
    video development, 70, 71
DiMaL project, 59
Document-based diagnosis, 10
Domain concepts and strategies, 9
Domain-specific competences, 143
domain-specific learning activities, 64
Drawing conclusions, 67, 74
Dyspnea, 113

E
Educational decisions, 64
Educational research, 50
Educational systems, 34
Effectiveness, 50
E-learning, 114
Empirical evidence, 10
Epistemic activities, 67
Epistemic-diagnostic activities, 19
Error situations, 19
Evaluating evidence, 75
Evidence evaluation, 19, 67
Evidence generation, 19
Expert-novice comparison, 75
Explanation, 51, 58, 66, 67

F
Face-to-face role-plays, 6
Familiarization, 133
Fiction contract, 54
Four-point Likert scale, 43

H
Heterogeneity, 12, 13
Heuristic strategies, 36
High-density interaction, 34
Higher education, 98, 99
History-taking
    cooperation with other projects, 116
    essential diagnostic situation,
        physicians, 109
    instructional support measures, 110
    live simulations, 115, 118
    medical diagnoses, 110
    medical interview
        definition, 110
        diagnostic competences, 111, 112, 118
        model, 110
    physician-centered approach, 118
    research questions, 113, 118, 119
    role-plays, 118
    simulation
        design, 113, 114
        development, 113, 114

History-taking (cont.)
  simulation-based learning
         and assessment
      computer-based simulations, 112
      live simulations, 112
      role-plays, 112
      standardized patients, 112
      video simulations, 112
    standardized patients, 114, 116, 117
    test design and development, 115, 116
    validation process, 116–118
    video simulations, 115, 118
Holistic, real-world problems, 51
Hypothetico-deductive approach, 67

I
Identify indicators, 2
Identifying problems, 67
Ill-structured problems, 5
Individual diagnostic activities, 126
Individual learners' characteristics, 8
Individual learning
         prerequisites block, 6
Inductive approach, 67
Information, 2, 34
Inquiry learning tasks, 87
Instructional approach, 29
Instructional methods, 98
Instructional quality in biology lessons
  biology-specific features, 68
  classroom management, 68
  error-tolerant classroom
         culture, 68
  scientific reasoning, 68
  subject-specific features, 68
  teaching effectiveness, 67
Instructional support, 6, 110, 119, 145
Integration, 51
Intelligent systems, 98
Interaction-based diagnosis, 10
Interdisciplinary
         collaborations, 87–89
Interdisciplinary commonalities, 1
Interdisciplinary research, 147
Internal collaboration scripts, 129
Interdisciplinary collaboration, 76
Interviewees' statements, 75

J
Joint conceptual framework, 2
Judgment accuracy, 50, 51

K
Knowledge acquisition, 65
Knowledge domains, 51
Knowledge forms, 18
Knowledge of learning processes, 52
Knowledge structures, 69
Knowledge test, 24
Knowledge types, 24

L
Learning competences, 98
Learning environment, 102
Learning opportunity, 87, 88
Learning phase, 101
Learning scenario, 53
Live simulations, 112, 117, 119

M
Mathematical argumentation skills
  central learning goal, 36
  diagnostic situation, 36
  prerequisites, 36
  proof-based science, 36
Mathematical competence levels model, 20
Mathematical competence model, 21, 29
Mathematical content knowledge, 36, 37
Mathematical problems, 28
Mathematical thinking, 57
Mathematics, 36
Mathematics education, 2
Medical education, 1, 2, 52, 124
Medical interview
  definition, 110
  diagnostic competences, 111, 112, 118
  model, 110
Medical research, 19
Medical/educational decisions, 98
Medicine/text comprehension problems, 2
Meta-analysis
  aim, 11
  empirical studies, 11, 13
  problem-solving process, 11
  professional knowledge, 11
  research questions, 12
  simulation effects, 12
Meta-analytic studies, 6
Metacognitive prompts, 10
Metacognitive strategies, 36
Meta-knowledge, 128
Methodological knowledge, 36, 37
Micro-teaching events, 56

Misconceptions
  arithmetic, 22
  competence areas, 20
  place value, 20
  primary students, 22
  specific topic area, 19
  students' mathematical, 24
  systematic errors, 20
  virtual students, 23, 24
Modeling complex problems, 20
Moderation effects, 59

N
National teacher training standards, 18
Natural language processing
          (NLP) methods, 98, 103
Nediko group, 19
Novices, 52
Numbers and operations, 21, 22

O
Observer Research Tool, 76
One-on-one diagnostic interviews
  derived measures, 57
  diagnostic situation, 53
  mastering professional demands, 58
  materials development, 55–56
  phases, 54–55
  scenarios, 53
  training actors, 56, 57

P
Participants' individual prerequisites, 44
Patient-centered medical interviews, 110
Patterns and structures, 21, 22
Pedagogical content knowledge
          (PCK), 18, 20, 34, 51, 65
Pedagogical decision, 50
Pedagogical interventions, 51
Pedagogical knowledge (PK), 18, 20, 65
Physician-centered interviews, 110
Polarizing filter, 90
Predictions, 51, 66, 67
Pre-service teachers
  automatic adaptive feedback, 104
  automation, 105
  communication with students, 24
  competence level selection, 25
  competence-oriented learning, 105
  diagnostic competences, 29
  diagnostic processes, 27, 28, 44
  diagnostic skills, 34, 35
  education, 59
  epistemic activities, 104
  feedback description, 102, 103
  final diagnosis, 27
  high-density interactions, 34
  higher education, 98, 99
  interdisciplinary setting, 100, 101
  learning environment, 27
  mathematical problems classification, 28
  medical education, 104
  NLP algorithms, 103
  nonadaptive feedback, 104
  observations, 26
  professional knowledge, 59
  ratings, 43
  real classroom situations, 35
  simulated environment, 27, 35
  simulation, 101, 102
  simulation-based learning, 105
  student selection, 25
  teachers' diagnosing, 99, 100
  titles, 25
  types of feedback, 104
  virtual student's misconception, 27
Problem-based learning approach, 12
Problem-solving and reasoning, 1
Problem-solving strategies, 36, 37
Professional actors, 114
Professional collaboration
          knowledge, 128–130
Professional competencies, 2
Professional knowledge, 7, 8, 51, 64, 128
Professional vision, 66, 75
Prompts, 9, 10, 69
Proof scheme, 36
Proof structure, 36
Propositional knowledge, 18
Psychological disorders, 99

Q
Qualitative evaluations, 50
Quality of diagnoses, 130

R
Real-life diagnostic situations, 144
Real-world classroom, 44
Reasoning skills, 66
Reflection, 10, 12
Research questions, 29

Role-play-based simulations
  approximations of practice, 58
  diagnostic interview, 54
  diagnostic situation, 54
  fostering communicative
    competences, 52
  medical education, 52
  one-on-one interviews (*see* One-on-one
    diagnostic interviews)
  screening tasks, 54
Role-taking, 10

S
Scaffolding
  complex cognitive skills
    development, 9
  definition, 9
  prompts, 9
  reflection, 10
  role-taking, 10
Scaffolding procedures, 5
Science teacher education, 66
Scientific discovery as dual search
  model (SDDS), 126
Scientific reasoning skills, 68
Screening tasks, 55, 57
Scripted videos, 35
  selection of practice, 37, 38
  student–teacher interactions, 37
  video production, 39
  vignette script development, 39
Self-explanation prompts, 10
Self-regulation, 12
Simulated learning environment
  development
  case knowledge, 21
  competence areas, 21, 22
  higher competence levels, 23
  mathematical competence model, 21
  mathematical problems, 21, 23
  problem selection process, 22, 23
  students' mathematical
    competences diagnosis, 21
  VERA-3 pilot studies, 22
  VERA-3 solutions, 23
  virtual third graders, 21, 23
Simulation, 87, 88
  practice authentic cases, 9
  central goal, 6
  characteristics, 6
  effectiveness, 6
  generalizability, 6

Simulation-based learning, 98, 119
  approximation of practice, 1
  effectiveness, 1
  empirical research, 11
  environments, 3
  support forms, 9
Simulations in higher education
  adaptability, 146
  diagnostic activities, 144
  future contributions, 147
  instructional support, learning
    diagnostic competences, 145
  learners, 145, 146
  medical domain, 143
  real-life diagnostic, 144
  scaffolding, 146
  teacher education, 143
Situational and social dependencies, 66
Situation-specific skills, 64
  conceptualizations, 66
  diagnosing classroom situations, 66, 67
  diagnosing context, 66
  evaluating evidence, 67
  individual characteristics, 66
  mediator, 66
  professional vision, 66
  reasoning skills, 66, 67
Social skills, 125
Socio-mathematical norms, 36
Standardization, 53
Standardization study, 23
Strategic knowledge, 7, 18, 111, 116, 128
Structured report format, 56
Student's mathematical
  learning status, 26, 28
Students' competence level, 28
Students' knowledge
  and misconceptions, 56
Students' learning progress, 18
Students' mathematical thinking, 50
Students' psychological problems, 99, 100
Student-teacher interactions, 34, 36, 50, 51

T
Task Alternative Strategy, 74
Task *Describe*, 72
Teacher education, 1, 2, 51, 98–100, 105
Teacher training, 18
Teacher's knowledge, 18
Teachers' diagnostic competences, 18
Teachers' diagnostic judgments, 18
Teachers' diagnostic skills, 37

Teachers' domain-specific
    knowledge schemas, 65
Teachers' expertise, 68
Teachers' professional development, 64
Teachers' professional knowledge
  diagnostic competences, 65
  domain-specific knowledge schemas, 65
  facets, 65
  instructional quality, 65
  teaching experience, 65
  teaching strategies, 65
Teacher–student dialogue, 36
Teaching performance, 64
Technical familiarization, 42
Technical knowledge, 20
Test performance block, 6
Theoretical and empirical research, 12
Theoretical framework, 12
Traditional paper-and-pencil-based
    assessments, 59
Typical errors, 20

U
University-based teacher education, 51, 53
University education, 64
University teacher education, 34

V
Validation process, 116–118, 135, 136
Van Hiele's model of children's
    development, 37
VERA-3 pilot studies, 22
Video-based implementation, 59
Video-based instruments, 69
Video-based simulation
  complexity reduction, 44
  conceptualization, 44
  design, 40–43
  empirical analyses, 43
  guiding questions, 37
  pre-service teachers' diagnostic
    skills development, 43
  real-world mathematics classrooms, 43
  scripted videos, 37–39, 43
Video-based simulations, 69
  accuracy, 92
  biology, 85
  cognitive and context-specific
    performance, 85

  cognitive skills, 85
  collaborative diagnosing, 88
  content-related facets, 92
  control of variables strategy, 84
  cross-curricular/cross-domain
    skills, 84
  cross-domain skills, 84, 85, 88
  developing video scripts, 90
  developmental psychology, 85
  diagnostic activities, 85
  diagnostic competences, 86
  domain, 85
  domain-general, 85
  efficiency, 92
  environment, 92
  exemplifying domain, 84
  formulation of hypotheses, 84
  inquiry tasks, 88
  interaction, 90
  interface, 89, 90
  learning opportunity, 87, 88
  material, 90
  performance evaluation, 92
  physics, 85
  planning and documentation
    phases, 90
  platform, 89
  pre-service teachers, 88
  scientific reasoning, 84, 86, 87
  segment of reality, 88
  segments, 91
  skills, 84
  students, 86
  subject-specific knowledge, 84
  teachers professional knowledge, 85
  teachers diagnostic competences, 85
  types, 92
  types of knowledge, 85
Videos
  authentic insights, 35
  professional teacher
    education medium, 35
  scripted video format, 35
  student-teacher interactions, 35
Video simulations, 112, 117
Vignette script development, 39

W
Web-based learning, 98
Web-based simulation environment, 55

The manufacturer's authorised representative in the EU is Springer Nature Customer Service Centre GmbH, Europaplatz 3, 69115 Heidelberg, Germany. If you have any concerns regarding our products, please contact ProductSafety@springernature.com

Printed and bound by CPI Group (UK) Ltd, Croydon, CR0 4YY

23/03/2026

02076380-0009